JAK Inhibitors in
Dermatology

Cover page represents the CD4 cell lines and a depictive diagram of the JAK receptor.

JAK Inhibitors in **Dermatology**

Editor

Kabir Sardana
MD DNB MNAMS
Director-Professor and Head
Department of Dermatology
Dr Ram Manohar Lohia Hospital and
Atal Bihari Vajpayee Institute of Medical Sciences (ABVIMS)
New Delhi, India

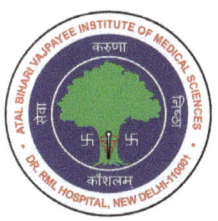

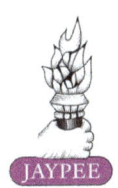

JAYPEE
JAYPEE BROTHERS MEDICAL PUBLISHERS
The Health Sciences Publisher
New Delhi | London

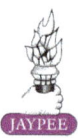 **Jaypee Brothers Medical Publishers (P) Ltd**

Headquarters
EMCA House
23/23-B, Ansari Road, Daryaganj
New Delhi 110 002, India
Landline: +91-11-23272143, +91-11-23272703
+91-11-23282021, +91-11-23245672
E-mail: jaypee@jaypeebrothers.com

Corporate Office
Jaypee Brothers Medical Publishers (P) Ltd.
4838/24, Ansari Road, Daryaganj
New Delhi 110 002, India
Phone: +91-11-43574357
Fax: +91-11-43574314
E-mail: jaypee@jaypeebrothers.com

Overseas Office
JP Medical Ltd.
83, Victoria Street, London
SW1H 0HW (UK)
Phone: +44-20 3170 8910
Fax: +44(0)20 3008 6180
E-mail: info@jpmedpub.com

EU GPSR Authorised Representative
LOGOS EUROPE, 9 rue Nicolas Poussin
17000, LA ROCHELLE, France
Phone: +33 (0) 6 67 93 73 78
Email: Contact@logos europe.eu

Website: www.jaypeebrothers.com
Website: www.jaypeedigital.com

© 2024, Jaypee Brothers Medical Publishers

The views and opinions expressed in this book are solely those of the original contributor(s)/author(s) and do not necessarily represent those of editor(s) or publisher of the book.

All rights reserved. No part of this publication may be reproduced, stored or transmitted in any form or by any means, electronic, mechanical, photocopying, recording or otherwise, without the prior permission in writing of the publishers.

All brand names and product names used in this book are trade names, service marks, trademarks or registered trademarks of their respective owners. The publisher is not associated with any product or vendor mentioned in this book.

Medical knowledge and practice change constantly. This book is designed to provide accurate, authoritative information about the subject matter in question. However, readers are advised to check the most current information available on procedures included and check information from the manufacturer of each product to be administered, to verify the recommended dose, formula, method and duration of administration, adverse effects and contraindications. It is the responsibility of the practitioner to take all appropriate safety precautions. Neither the publisher nor the author(s)/editor(s) assume any liability for any injury and/or damage to persons or property arising from or related to use of material in this book.

This book is sold on the understanding that the publisher is not engaged in providing professional medical services. If such advice or services are required, the services of a competent medical professional should be sought.

Every effort has been made where necessary to contact holders of copyright to obtain permission to reproduce copyright material. If any have been inadvertently overlooked, the publisher will be pleased to make the necessary arrangements at the first opportunity.

Inquiries for bulk sales may be solicited at: jaypee@jaypeebrothers.com

JAK Inhibitors in Dermatology / **Kabir Sardana**

First Edition: **2024**

ISBN: 978-93-5696-564-5

> *"He who has a why to live can bear almost any how"*
> Viktor Frankel quoting Nietzsche in "Man Search for Meaning"

This concept called "Logotherapy" was developed by psychologist Viktor Frankl in response to the unspeakable horrors of a Nazi death camp in which he was held captive during the Holocaust. He survived unimaginable horrors, and in the crucible of suffering he came to the realization that the human spirit is such that it can endure anything if given a reason, any reason, to do so.

Find a reason "why" to live and the "how" will follow. The "why" to live can be love of an idea, or of a project you want to accomplish or maybe something else.

The "why" you find is called hope. And the "how" which finds itself is the defeat of despair. Find within yourself the "why", and the "how" will find itself!

Contributors

Amrutha Solanke MBBS
Senior Resident
Department of Dermatology
Goa Medical College
Goa, India

Ananta Khurana MD DNB MNAMS FRCP (L)
Professor
Department of Dermatology
Dr Ram Manohar Lohia Hospital and
Atal Bihari Vajpayee Institute of Medical
Sciences (ABVIMS)
New Delhi, India

Anupam Das MD
Assistant Professor
Department of Dermatology
KPC Medical College and Hospital
Kolkata, West Bengal, India

Debatri Datta MD
Consultant Dermatologist
Oliva Skin and Hair Clinic
Kolkata, West Bengal, India

Gautam Kumar Singh MD
Professor
Department of Dermatology
Bharati Vidyapeeth (Deemed to be
University) Medical College and Hospital
Pune, Maharashtra, India

Jaspriya Sandhu MD DNB MNAMS
Associate Professor
Department of Dermatology,
Venereology and Leprology
Dayanand Medical College and Hospital
Ludhiana, Punjab, India

Kabir Sardana MD DNB MNAMS
Director-Professor and Head
Department of Dermatology
Dr Ram Manohar Lohia Hospital
and Atal Bihari Vajpayee Institute of
Medical Sciences (ABVIMS)
New Delhi, India

Kittu Malhi MD
Assistant Professor
Department of Dermatology,
Venereology and Leprology
Dayanand Medical College and Hospital
Ludhiana, Punjab, India

Prasanna Duraisamy MBBS MD FRGUHS
Consultant Dermatologist
Department of Dermatology
Universal Hospital
Erode, Tamil Nadu, India

Ramkumar Ramamoorthy MD
Consultant Pediatric Dermatologist
Department of Dermatology
Kanchi Kamakoti Child's Trust Hospital
Chennai, Tamil Nadu, India

Shikha Shah MD DNB
Senior Resident
Department of Dermatology,
Venereology and Leprology
Postgraduate Institute of Medical
Education and Research (PGIMER)
Chandigarh, India

Shivani Bansal MD DNB MNAMS
Assistant Professor
Department of Dermatology
All India Institute of Medical Sciences (AIIMS)
Bathinda, Punjab, India

Soumya Jagadeesan MD
Professor
Department of Dermatology
Amrita Institute of Medical Sciences
Kochi, Tamil Nadu, India

Sunil Dogra MD DNB FAAD FRCP(London) FRCP(Edinburgh)
Professor
Department of Dermatology, Venereology and Leprology
Postgraduate Institute of Medical Education and Research (PGIMER)
Chandigarh, India

Sushama Sushama MD
Senior Resident
Department of Dermatology
All India Institute of Medical Sciences (AIIMS)
Bathinda, Punjab, India

Varadraj V Pai MD
Assistant Professor
Department of Dermatology
Goa Medical College
Goa, India

Preface

Are JAK inhibitors the new steroid?

This book "*JAK Inhibitors in Dermatology*" and its contents were part of the previous book *Systemic Drugs in Dermatology*, and even at that time this class of drugs seemed to be a revolutionary addition to the tools we employ to treat patients. Unlike theorists and scientists we have the advantage of using drugs and biologicals. Outside of conference talks in real world biologicals across the board except for omalizumab and rituximab have not been a great boon as the "goal post" of cytokine inhibition keeps shifting, and I speak out of extensive usage of these drugs at RMLH. The sponsored conference talks that we have little long-term data to support their professed knowledge and the "In my experience…." dictum is the most lame scientific logic, especially as most may have a follow-up of a few months. The fact that a revolution has occurred in cytokine profiling shows that even the common, much "talked of disease" psoriasis is not a monocytokine disease. That itself is proof of how inane is the biological industries professed cure or efficacy of biologicals!

At the other end of the spectrum is the inane, illogical, and dogmatic use of steroids, especially the self-styled "magical" pulse regimens that have outlived their life of logic! This is important to appreciate as these "pulse regimens" are written by many of us and in times of medicolegal scrutiny should be discarded. The genesis of my interest was after a index case of alopecia totalis who also has juvenile idiopathic arthritis (JIA) and had gone through multiple treatments, including, dexamethasone cyclophosphamide pulse (DCP) and pulse dexamethasone and was told by two institutes that nothing can be done, was put on tofacitinib. Not only did she get all her hair back in 2019, she is still on the drug with a maintenance of the hair growth. There have been no side effects to date (after 5 years) and also highlights the need for maintenance dose regimens and the need to examine the T memory cells.

To understand Janus kinase (JAK) inhibitors one needs to have a working knowledge of basic immunology. Unlike many speakers who claim to be experts, with zero research data, at our institute, every alternate thesis is an aspect of immunology. And that includes individual cells like Treg cells and memory T cells, cytokines both in serum and skin and STAT (signal transducer and activator of transcription)/JAK receptors. This helps as we know the difference between "talking the walk" and "walking the talk". This data is then used to generate therapeutic data; this is the reason that the book begins with basic and applied immunology. These sections would help the reader understand why and how to predict JAK usage. We have then covered the varied approved and unapproved usages followed by monitoring protocols and side effects.

For many years we have been prescribing steroids varied pulses and also DCP, in an arbitrary, dogmatic pattern. DCP may have been necessary in its era, but each aspect of this, derived from the lupus nephritis protocol of National Institute of Health (NIH), is arbitrary, and there is no logic in repeated arbitrary suppression of all the immune cells both by intravenous (IV) and oral cyclophosphamide. This is the era of specific targeted therapy and JAK inhibitors with their ability to target cytokine/s families with the advantage of oral usage, and their cost is a harbinger of a therapeutic revolution.

Finally, my grateful thanks to Shri Jitendar P Vij (Group Chairman), Mr Ankit Vij (Managing Director), Ms Chetna Malhotra (Senior Director—Professional Publishing, Marketing, and Business Development), Ms Pooja Bhandari (Director—Production), Ms Himani Pandey (Development Editor), Ms Seema Dogra (Cover Visualizer), Mr Nitin Bhardwaj (Senior Graphic Designer) and the entire Production and Designing Team of M/s Jaypee Brothers Medical Publishers (P) Ltd, New Delhi, India for their valuable contribution and incredible support.

It's time to look beyond steroids and look at novel drugs like JAK inhibitor, and I hope the book helps you rewrite your prescription and dispel the notion that dermatologists have just one tool in their basket steroids.

Kabir Sardana

Contents

1. **Immunology: Basics and Applied**   1
   Kabir Sardana

2. **Cytokines Signaling Pathway and Role of JAK-STAT Pathway**   19
   Kabir Sardana

3. **JAK Inhibitors: An Overview**   31
   Kabir Sardana

4. **JAK Inhibitors in Alopecia Areata**   46
   Debatri Datta, Anupam Das

5. **JAK Inhibitors in Atopic Dermatitis**   55
   Kittu Malhi, Jaspriya Sandhu

6. **JAK Inhibitor in Psoriasis: Looking beyond Biologicals**   68
   Kabir Sardana

7. **Janus Kinase Inhibitors in Vitiligo**   73
   Shivani Bansal, Sushama Sushama

8. **JAK Inhibitors for Eczematous Conditions**   82
   Soumya Jagadeesan, Prasanna Duraisamy

9. **JAK Inhibitors in Pruritic Disorders**   90
   Ramkumar Ramamoorthy, Kabir Sardana

10. **Off-label Uses of Janus Kinase Inhibitors**   96
    Kabir Sardana

11. **Adverse Effects of JAK Inhibitors**   111
    Varadraj V Pai, Amrutha Solanke

12. **Baseline Tests and Monitoring**   125
    Ananta Khurana

13. **Common Janus Kinase Inhibitor Drugs**   133
    Kabir Sardana, Sunil Dogra, Shikha Shah

Index   143

CHAPTER 1

Immunology: Basics and Applied

Kabir Sardana

"It's never too late – never too late to start over, never too late to be happy."
—Jane Fonda

Overview

- Introduction
- Overview
- Overview of Innate and Adaptive Immune Response
- Antigen Presentation and Activation of Immune Response
- Cytokine Receptors and Signaling
- Which are the Main Subsets and Functions of T Lymphocytes?
- Lymphocyte and Cytokine Interaction and Regulation of the Immune System
- Where do JAKs Come into the Picture?

■ INTRODUCTION

Immunology is often a topic that is not studied in medical college or in formal dermatology training, which is unfortunate, as this forms the basis for understanding many autoimmune and inflammatory disease and applied uses of various drugs in a host of autoimmune disorders. Probably a lack of knowledge of this aspect is the reason why most clinicians persist with the use of steroids or immunosuppressive drugs, which usually have a more pervasive suppression of bystander immune and nonimmune cells and leading to widespread adverse events. Thus as the quote in the header of the chapter states, its never too late to start reading.

Janus kinase inhibitors (JAKinibs) represent a class of drugs that are <u>highly specific</u> in action as they target one type of signal transmitters, which make their effect targeted and more focused than steroids and immunosuppressive agent (ISA). It is thus important to understand the basics of immunology, so that one can appreciate where JAKinibs work and how we can predict disorders where this class of drugs can be used successfully.

■ OVERVIEW

Immunity is divided into two discrete parts which can occasionally overlap:
1. The first is the **innate** (or natural), which is composed of salient cells including, macrophages, dendritic cells (DCs), granulocytes (neutrophils, basophils, and eosinophils), natural killer (NK) cells, the complement system, and acute phase proteins.

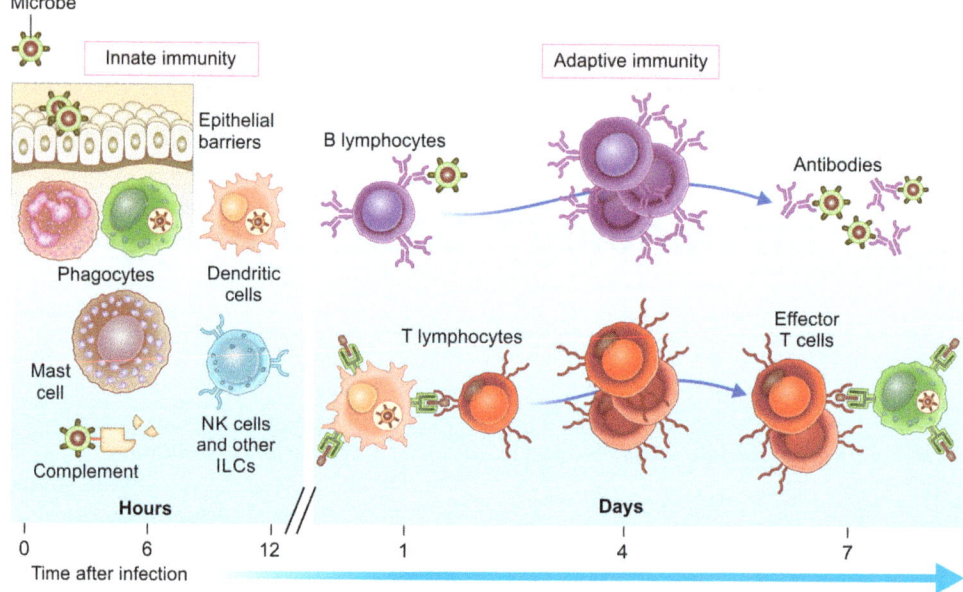

(ILCs: innate lymphoid cells; NK: natural killer)

FIG. 1: Innate and adaptive immunity. The mechanisms of innate immunity provide the initial defense against infections. Adaptive immune responses develop later and require the activation of lymphocytes. The kinetics of the innate and adaptive immune responses may vary in different infections.

2. The **adaptive response**, mediated by B and T cells (**Fig. 1**) is usually relevant to most disease processes.

The immune cells express sensors which are known as **"pathogen-associated molecular pattern receptors"** (PAMPRs), also known as pattern recognition receptors (PRRs), and damage-associated molecular pattern receptors (DAMPRs), which identify foreign antigens and help to mount defense against them. Thus, the end result is that the natural immunity cells provide first line of defense, and usually successful in eliminating pathogens and also help to prime the adaptive immune system if the innate immunity is unable to control the antigen influx. This is much like the paramilitary forces that acts the first defense and the army that acts as the major defense of a country.

The **sensors** of B and T cells are the antigen receptors [membrane immunoglobulins and T-cell receptors (TCRs), respectively], which are dissimilar to each other in terms of specificity; each receptor recognizes one antigen and especially a few peptide residues on it (epitope). However, by taking as a whole the pool of lymphocytes, their receptors offer a vast array of specificities that are more than the genes of the human body. As a unique singular rearrangement for each peptide chain of the receptor is allowed, thus the immune cells retain their antigenic specificity. The intercellular *communication* is by cell-to-cell contact using adhesion molecules or by soluble mediators known as cytokines or chemokines.

Central (taking place in bone marrow and thymus) and peripheral (taking place in the lymph nodes) *tolerance* is essential, so that the immune system does not attack the host systems and a loss of this tolerance leads to autoimmunity.

The role of **JAKi** lies in the cell-to-cell interaction via cytokines, and hence, we will focus on the adaptive immune response, which is largely mediated by the T lymphocytes.

■ OVERVIEW OF INNATE AND ADAPTIVE IMMUNE RESPONSE

Notably, while the initial response to an antigenic stimuli is via innate immunity, the late response is by the adaptive immunity. Adaptive immunity is specific for different microbial and nonmicrobial antigens and is increased by repeated exposures to antigen (immunologic memory).

Lymphocytes are the main cells that mediate adaptive immunity. Of the many cell lines, there are various clades with unique cytokines that premediate effector action. The major subsets of lymphocytes are B and T cells

The *adaptive immune response* is initiated by the recognition of foreign antigens. Specialized antigen-presenting cells (APCs) capture the foreign antigen, and the antigenic components are then recognized by the target lymphocytes. There are subtypes of lymphocytes, which help to act on the foreign antigen leading to release of effector cytokines. This is followed by the formation of memory cells. These cells are useful for enhanced response in case of an encounter of the antigenic stimuli on subsequent encounters.

Humoral immunity is mediated by antibodies secreted by B lymphocytes and the subtypes including plasma cells and helps to contain extracellular microbes. These antibodies help to eliminate the infectivity of microbes and also promote the elimination of microbes by phagocytes and by activation of the complement system (**Fig. 1**).

Cell-mediated immunity is mediated by T lymphocytes and cytokines and work against intracellular microbes. The CD4+ helper T lymphocytes with the help of macrophages eliminate ingested microbes and also stimulate B cells to produce antibodies. CD8+ cytotoxic T lymphocytes (CTLs) kill cells harboring intracellular pathogens, thus eliminating reservoirs of infection (**Fig. 1**).

■ ANTIGEN PRESENTATION AND ACTIVATION OF IMMUNE RESPONSE

The antigen receptors of most T cells recognize only peptides displayed by major histocompatibility complex (MHC) molecules on the surface of APCs. **CD4+** helper T lymphocytes recognize antigens in association with class II MHC molecules while the **CD8+** CTLs recognize antigens when presented with class I MHC molecules.

The APCs capture and process the antigen and activate the T cells. DCs are the most efficient APCs for initiating primary responses and activate the naive T cells, and macrophages and B lymphocytes and present antigens to helper T cells in the effector phase of cell-mediated immunity and in humoral immune responses, respectively (**Fig. 2**).

Dendritic cells capture antigens from their sites of entry (epithelial lining) or production (in lymphoid tissues) and transport these antigens to secondary (peripheral) lymphoid organs. Naive T cells that recirculate through these organs recognize the antigens, and primary immune responses are induced in these organs. Notably most of the action of immune cells is mediated by cytokines.

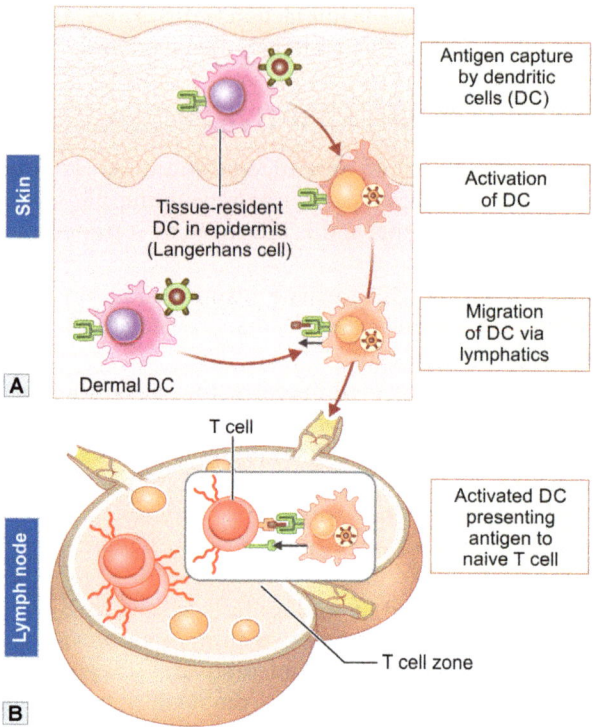

FIGS. 2A AND B: A schematic diagram that shows the process of antigen capture by skin resident dendritic cells which then migrate via the lymphatics and activate the naive T cells in the lymph node.

■ CYTOKINE RECEPTORS AND SIGNALING

Cytokine signals through receptors.[1] We will detail the salient cytokines as they form the basis of JAK inhibitors.

Classes of Cytokine Receptors

The most widely used classification of cytokine receptors is based on structural homologies of the extracellular cytokine-binding domains and shared intracellular signaling mechanisms (**Fig. 3**).

Type I Cytokine Receptors (Hematopoietin Receptor Family)

This class includes <u>short-chain cytokines</u> and have the common cytokine receptor γ-**chain** (γc) family [interleukin (IL-2), IL-4, IL-7, IL-9, IL-15, and IL-21] and, **thymic stromal lymphopoietin (TSLP)** and **IL-13**, the common β-**chain** *(βc)* family [IL-3, IL-5, and granulocyte-macrophage colony-stimulating factor (GM-CSF)], M-CSF and stem cell factor (SCF). The <u>long-chain cytokines</u> include the gp130 family (IL-6, IL-11, OSM, LIF, CNTF, CT1, and NNT1) as well as G-CSF, leptin, erythropoietin (EPO), thrombopoietin (TPO), growth hormone, and prolactin (PRL). The other cytokines include IL-2, IL-3, IL-6, IL-12, and IL-23 family, which play a role in psoriasis. All the type I cytokine receptors engage JAK-signal transducer and activator of transcription (**JAK-STAT**) signaling pathways, as discussed later (**Fig. 3B**).

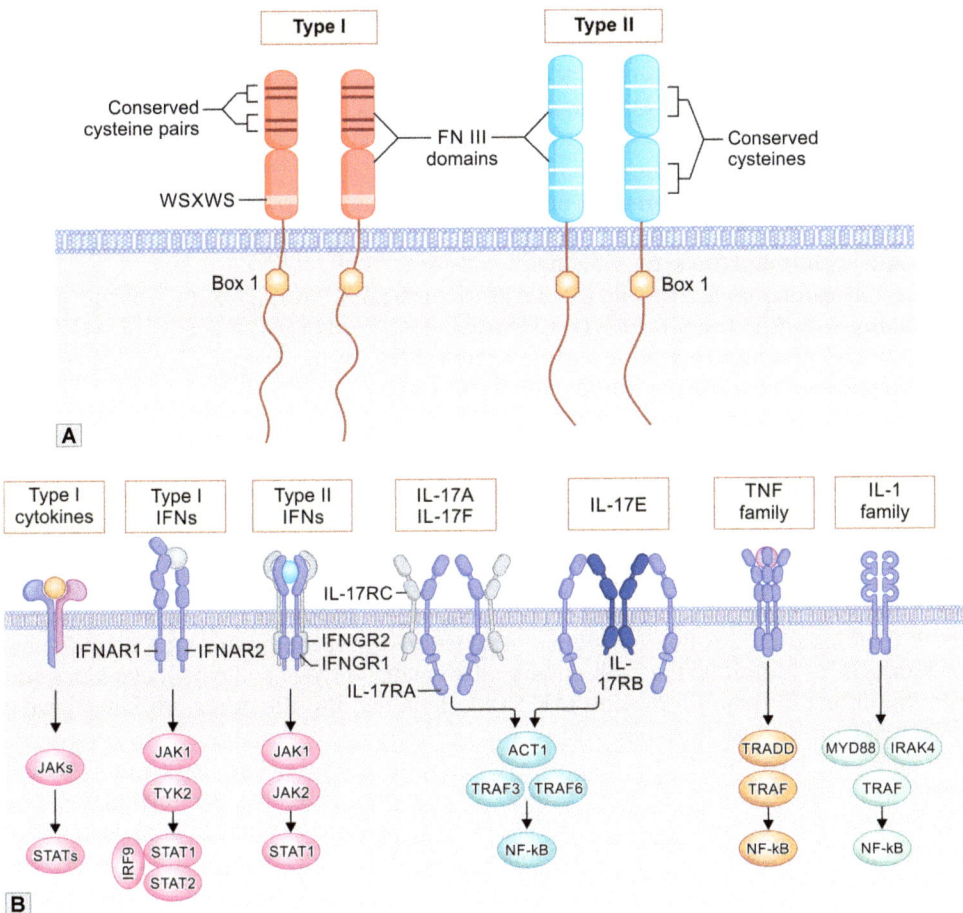

(IL: interleukin; JAK: Janus kinase; TNF: tumor necrosis factor)

FIGS. 3A AND B: (A) Type I cytokine receptor chains contain two fibronectin III (FN III) domains, with the N-terminal one containing two sets of conserved cysteines and the more proximal one a WSXWS motif. There is also a cytoplasmic 'Box 1' region for the binding of JAKs, so that they activate JAK–signal transducer and activator of transcription (JAK–STAT) signaling. Type II cytokine receptors also have a FN III domain, conserved cysteines, and a Box 1 motif. (B) Type 1 and type II cytokines mediate their action via the JAK STAT pathway unlike the IL-17, TNF, and IL-1 family.

Type II Cytokine Receptors (Interferon Receptor Family)

This includes type I, II, and III interferons (**IFNs**) as well as **IL-10** family cytokines (IL-10, IL-16, IL-19, IL-20, IL-22, IL-24, and IL-26) (**Fig. 3B**).

Type I cytokines are monomers (although IL-5 forms a homodimer), whereas type II cytokines including IFNs and IL-10 are homodimers. Both type I and type II cytokines use JAK–STAT as a major signaling pathway. SCF is distinctive in that it is a type I cytokine that acts not through a typical type I receptor but instead via Kit, a receptor tyrosine kinase.

Other Cytokine Families

These include the IL-1, IL-17, tumor necrosis factor (TNF), and transforming growth factor beta (TGF-β) families.

The **IL-1** family is constituted by IL-1 (IL-1α, IL-1β, IL-1Ra, and IL-33), IL-18 (IL-18 and IL-37), and IL-36 (IL-36α, IL-36β, IL-36γ, IL-36Ra, and IL-38) subfamilies. The cytokine IL-37 interacts with IL-18Rα and IL-1R8 (SIGIRR) and limits inflammation mediated by toll-like receptor (TLR)–IL-1, IL-18, IL-33, and IL-36. IL-38 also has broad anti-inflammatory effects and can counteract the effect of IL-1 family cytokines apart from inhibiting their action. Thus, *IL-37* and *IL-38* are anti-inflammatory cytokines.

In healthy individuals, expression of **IL-17** is restricted by barrier surfaces, including the skin, intestine, conjunctiva, gingiva, and vaginal mucosa. IL-17 also has an important roles in wound healing and tissue remodeling.

The **TNF family** includes TNF, LT, TWEAK, Fas ligand, TRAIL, OX40L, CD30L, 4-1BB ligand, BAFF, APRIL, RANKL, LIGHT, CD40 ligand, CD70, TL1, GITR ligand, EDA-A1, and EDA-A2. TNF and its receptor form trimers and exhibit distinctive signaling mechanisms, including the activation of nuclear factor-κB (NF-κB).

Cytokine Receptors

Type I cytokines typically bind to homodimeric or heterodimeric receptors. For example, growth hormone is a monomeric cytokine that binds to a homodimer of the growth hormone receptor, which is a type I cytokine receptor (type I cytokine receptors are also known as hematopoietin receptors). Notably, within the cytoplasmic domain, there is a loci known as 'Box 1' that mediates recruitment of JAK family tyrosine kinases. Notably, the FN III domains and Box 1 regions are conserved in receptors for type II cytokines, including IFNs, indicating the evolutionary relationship of type I and type II cytokines and corresponding to them both using **JAK-STAT** signaling. But the other cytokines have a divergent receptor structures (Fig. 3A).

The **IL-17, TNF, and IL-1** families have different structures and use other signaling pathways (e.g., NF-κB) instead of JAK–STAT signaling (Fig. 3B). A knowledge of the cytokine families and their signaling via the JAK STAT pathway can help in predicting where JAKinib drugs can be used. Thus, disorders with a primary role of IL-17, IL-1, and TNF-α would not always respond to this class of drugs.

■ WHICH ARE THE MAIN SUBSETS AND FUNCTIONS OF T LYMPHOCYTES?[2]

Cell-mediated immunity is part of the adaptive immune response and is mediated by T lymphocytes and can be transferred from immunized to naive individuals by T cells. Naive CD4+ T lymphocytes may differentiate into different types of specialized effector T cells, in presence of cytokines. Thus, Th1 cells that secrete IFN-γ mediate defense against intracellular microbes; Th2 cells that secrete IL-4 and IL-5 favor immunoglobulin E (IgE) and eosinophil/mast cell-mediated immune reactions against helminths; Th17 cells that promote inflammation and mediate defense against extracellular fungi and bacteria (Fig. 4).

The above is a simplistic view, as now immunology of many dermatoses has proceeded beyond the three subtypes and a more detailed subtyping is useful (Fig. 5) for a comprehensive assessment of immunological cells.

- **CD3+ CD4– CD8– γδ T cells:** They serve as an early-stage defense mechanism in mucosal surfaces. The actual diversity of γδ TCR is very limited. They are triggered by alarm signals such as heat shock proteins and several metabolites of pathogenic bacteria. Some subsets of CD3+ CD4–CD8– γδ T cells do not require antigen presentation through MHC, resembling thus cells of the innate immune system. Their functions include tissue homeostasis and wound healing.

Effector T cells	Defining cytokines	Principal target cells	Major immune effect	Host defense	Role in disease
Th1	IFN-γ	Macrophages	Macrophage activation	Intracellular pathogens	Autoimmunity; chronic inflammation
Th2	IL-4 IL-5 IL-13	Eosinophils	Eosinophil and mast cell activation; alternative macrophage activation	Helminths	Allergy
Th17	IL-17 IL-22	Neutrophils	Neutrophil recruitment and activation	Extracellular bacteria and fungi	Autoimmunity; inflammation
Tfh	IL-21 (and IFN-γ or IL-4)	B cells	Antibody production	Extracellular pathogens	Autoimmunity (autoantibodies)

(IFN-γ: interferon gamma; IL: interleukin)

FIG. 4: Properties of the major subsets of CD4+ helper T cells. Naive CD4+ T cells may differentiate into distinct subsets of effector cells in response to antigen, costimulators, and cytokines. Each subset acts mainly on another cell of the immune system (referred to as target cells) and serves different functions and roles in disease.

- **CD8+ T cells:** CD4+ helper T cells promote naive CD8+ T-cell activation by several mechanisms (**Fig. 6**). These effector cells that are formed are known as 'cytotoxic T lymphocytes.' They recognize cells infected by viruses (target cells). The target cells express MHC class I molecules in complex with viral antigens and kill them via a process called apoptosis. CD8+ T cells in order to kill the target cell and reduce the burden of virus, release molecules such as perforins, granzymes, IFN-γ, and TNF-α and express on their surface Fas ligand (Fas-L) (**Fig. 7**). Perforins are molecules which penetrate the membrane of infected cells; they are polymerized making holes in the membrane, while granzymes pass through these holes and enter the target cell; within the target cell, granzymes activate the caspase cascade, which eventually leads to programmed cell death known as "apoptosis".
- **T helper (Th) 1 cells:** They recognize foreign antigens in complex with MHC class II molecules expressed on the surfaces of professional APCs. These cells contribute to killing of exclusively intracellular pathogens, such as bacteria entrapped into the phagosomes (*Mycobacterium tuberculosis*), as well as some viruses. The differentiation of naive T cells to Th1 phenotype is controlled by the cytokine IL-12. Cytokine signals combined with recognition of foreign antigens drive Th1 cells to secrete IFN-γ (**Fig. 5**). IFN-γ will stimulate phagocytes to fuse the phagosomes with the lysosomes making the so-called phagolysosomes.
- **Th2 cells:** They primarily stimulate immune responses against extracellular pathogens but also contribute to allergic reactions through stimulation of B cells. They provide help to certain B cells in order to produce IgE antibodies. They also secrete IL-4 and IL-13 (**Fig. 5**). Differentiation of Th2 cells largely depends on APCs, which produce IL-4 that differentiates naive T cells to the Th2 phenotype.
- **Regulatory T cells (Tregs):** These cells are generated when naive cells encounter antigen presented by cells that release TGF-β. These cells produce also TGF-β and IL-10

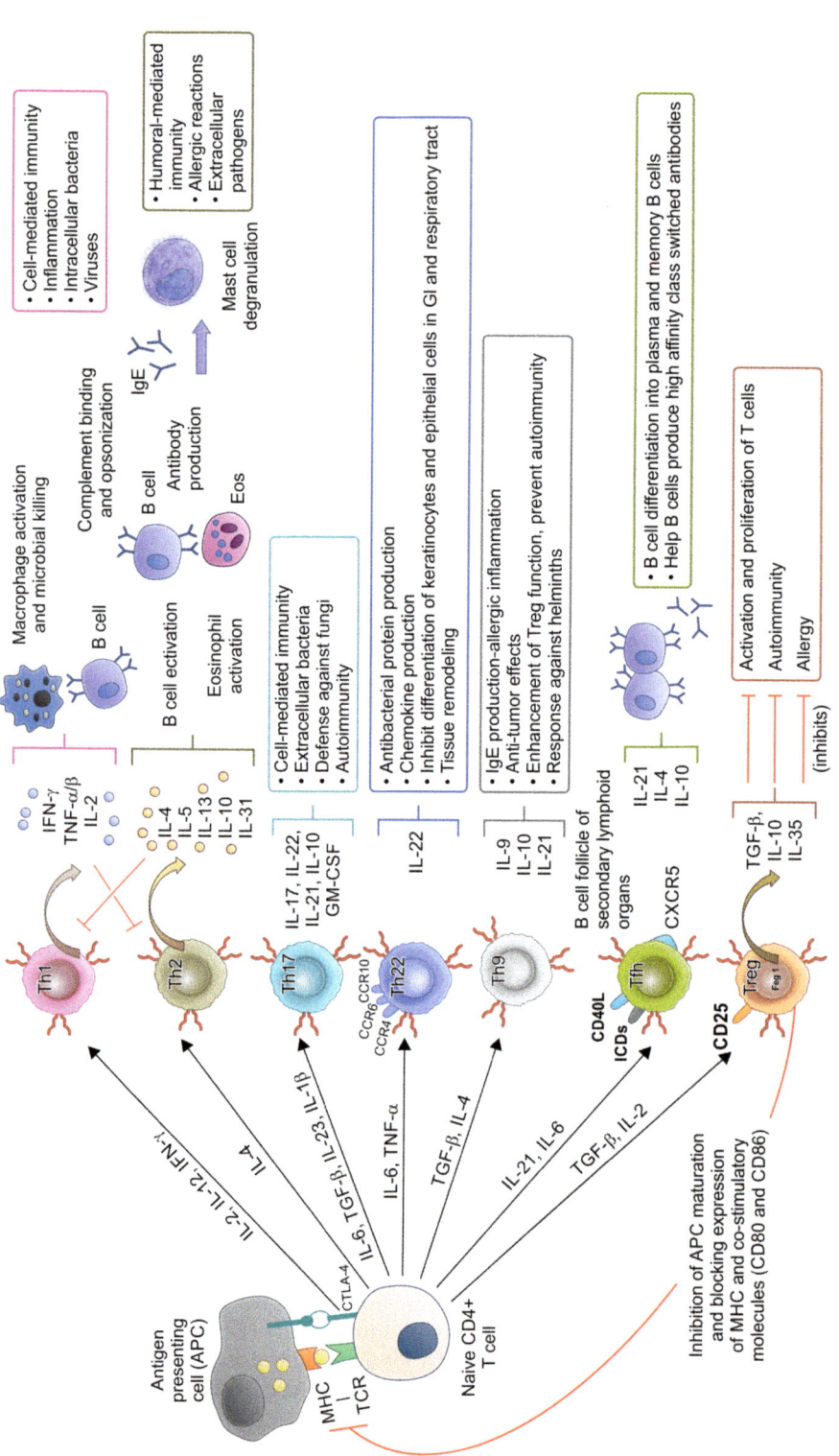

FIG. 5: The naive CD4 cell under the influence of cytokines can convert into varied CD4 cell types including Th1, Th2, Th17, Th22, Th9, and Tfh cell. Each of these releases effector cytokines which lead to cellular. The Treg cells serves to control the immune process and prevent unbridled and excessive stimulatory activity of varied cells lines.

(GM-CSF: granulocyte-macrophage colony-stimulating factor; IFN-γ: interferon gamma; IL: interleukin; MHC: major histocompatibility complex; TCR: T-cell receptor; TGF-β: transforming growth factor beta; TNF-α: tumor necrosis factor alpha)

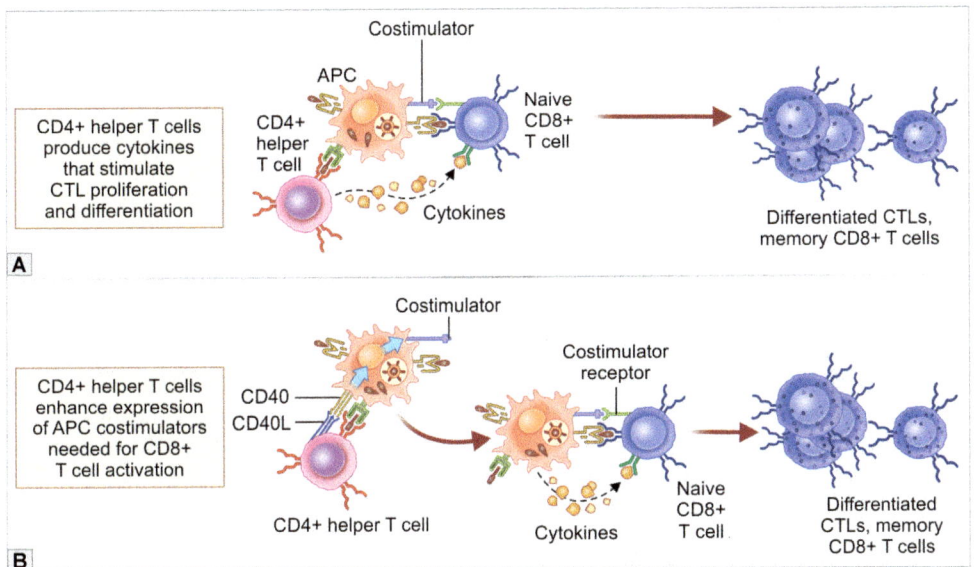

(APC: antigen-presenting cell; CTL: cytotoxic T lymphocyte)

FIGS. 6A AND B: CD4+ cells are help in the activation of CD8+ cells.

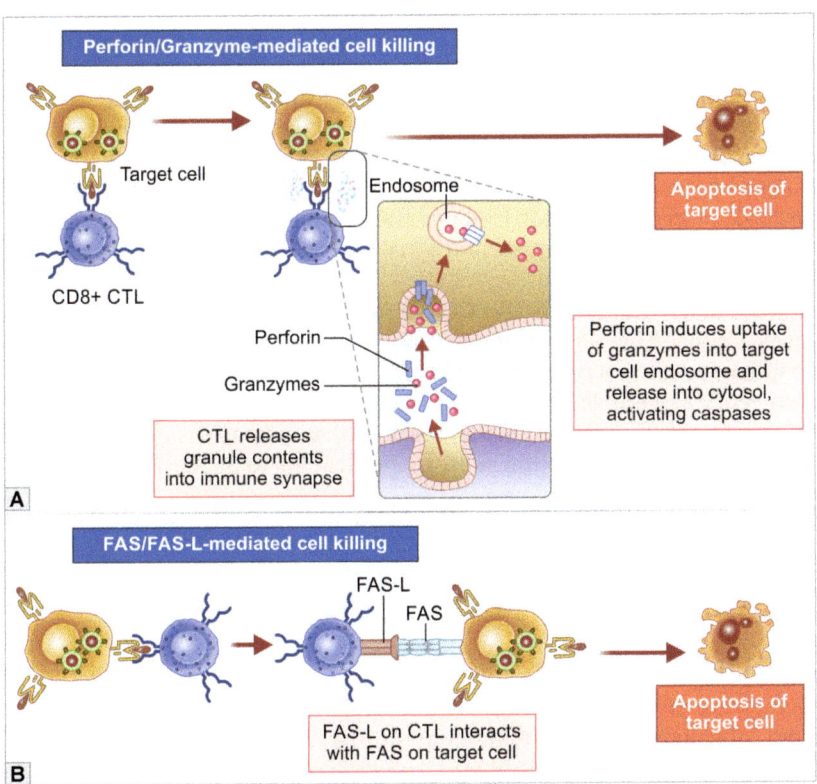

(CTL: cytotoxic T lymphocyte)

FIGS. 7A AND B: CD8 cells act by release of perforin/granzyme and cause FAS/FAS-L-mediated cell killing.

and downregulate immune responses. Tregs express CTL-associated protein 4 (CTLA-4) and CD25 molecules on their surface as well as the intracellular protein FOXP3, which is a transcription factor (Fig. 5). They function to control the aberrant cellular response.

- **Th17 cells:** These cells secrete IL-17, IL-22, and GM-CSF. They participate in surveillance of fungi and extracellular bacteria as well as in the maintenance of barrier integrity. However, Th17 cells can become a proinflammatory cell subpopulation. Th17 cells are generated by CD4+ naive T lymphocytes when they recognize an antigen expressed by a DC that produces TGF-β and IL-6. In addition to IL-6 and TGF-β, they are also stimulated by the cytokines IL-23 and IL-1β (Fig. 5). Th17 cells contribute to autoinflammatory diseases, such as rheumatoid arthritis, systemic lupus erythematosus, psoriasis, and multiple sclerosis.
- **T follicular helper (Tfh) cells:** These are CD4+ T cells found within B-cell follicles of secondary lymphoid organs. Tfh cells are identified by their B-cell follicle-homing receptor CXCR5, which is constitutively expressed on their surface. Tfh cells express CD40L and secrete IL-21 and IL-4. Using the above molecules, Tfh cells trigger the formation and maintenance of germinal centers and contribute to the differentiation of antigen-stimulated B cells to plasma cells in order to enhance antibody production (Fig. 5).
- **Th9 cells:** Th9 cells, a subset initially associated with the Th2 phenotype, are the primary source of IL-9. The production of IL-9 in Th9 cells is stimulated by TGF-β and IL-4 and inhibited by IFN-γ but seem to be capable of promoting allergic inflammation. Some of the effects of Th9 cells could be mediated through mast cells, but others are likely direct effects on tissue-resident cells. They play a role in infectious diseases, allergy, cancer, and autoimmune disorders.
- **Th22 cells:** Th22 cells are unique in that they express IL-22 but not IL-17 and IFN-γ, and express the master transcription factor aryl hydrocarbon receptor. In addition to the production of IL-22, Th22 cells are characterized by surface expression of the chemokine receptors CCR4, CCR6, and CCR10 that are associated with cutaneous T-cell homing. The major known functions of IL-22 are to regulate innate defense programs (e.g., antibacterial protein production), induce chemokine production, inhibit differentiation of some epithelial cells in the gastrointestinal and respiratory tracts, and stimulate tissue remodeling.

Notably, the differentiation of naive CD4+ T cells into subsets of helper T cells is induced by cytokines produced by APCs, by the T cells themselves and other cells. This is mediated by transcription factors that promote cytokine gene expression in the T cells and epigenetic changes in cytokine gene loci, which may be associated with stable commitment to a particular subset. Each subset produces cytokines that increase its own development and inhibit the development of the other subsets, thus leading to increasing polarization of the response.

■ LYMPHOCYTE AND CYTOKINE INTERACTION AND REGULATION OF THE IMMUNE SYSTEM[3]

CD4 Differentiation and Role of Cytokines[4]

As alluded to previously naive CD4+ T cells are able to differentiate into a variety of phenotypes, of which the prominent being the Th1, Th2, and Th17 phenotypes (Fig. 8), which are associated with type 1, type 2, and type 3 (which are sometimes also called

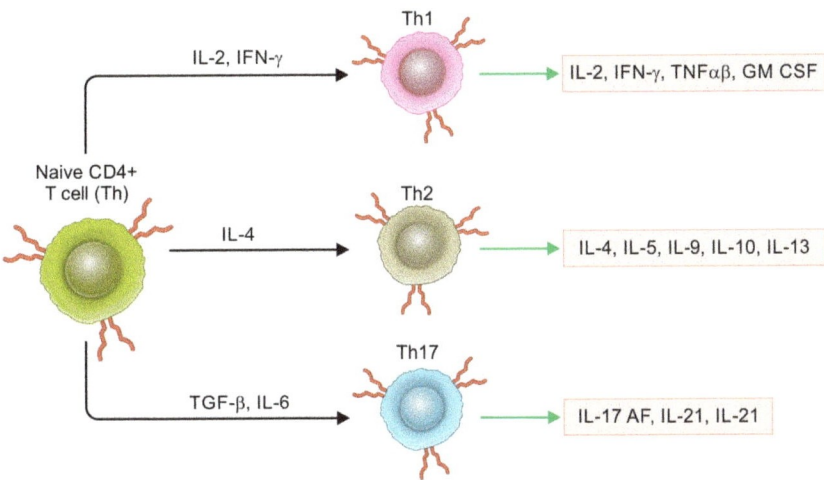

(IFN-γ: interferon gamma; GM-CSF: granulocyte–macrophage colony stimulating factor; TGF-β: transforming growth factor beta; TNF: tumor necrosis factor)

FIG. 8: Differentiation of murine Th cells. IL-12 and IFN-γ favor differentiation of Th1 cells, and IL-4 favors differentiation of Th2 cells. TGF-β and IL-6 drive Th17-cell development.

type 17) cytokine responses, respectively. This is crucial to the adaptive immune response. Varied factors that may influence the differentiation of Th cells include:
- The sites of antigen presentation
- Costimulatory molecules involved in cognate cellular interactions
- Peptide density and binding affinity–high MHC class II peptide density favors Th1 or Th17, low densities favor Th2
- APCs and the cytokines they produce
- The cytokine profile and balance of cytokines evoked by antigen
- Receptors expressed on the T cell
- Activity of costimulatory molecules and hormones present in the local environment
- Host genetic background, for example, some strains of mouse preferentially produce type 1 responses, while others tend to produce type 2 responses.

Cytokine Balance and Cross Regulation

There are important regulatory mechanisms that play a role in T-cell differentiation. Cytokines are part of an extracellular signaling network that plays a role to controls functions of the innate and adaptive immune system. The local cytokine milieu is heavily influenced by cytokines derived from innate immune cells in the early stages of an immune response. Cytokines and immune responses can be broadly classified as **type 1** (TH1), **type 2** (TH2), or **type 3** (sometimes called TH17).

Interleukin-12 is a potent initial stimulus for IFN-γ production by T cells and NK cells and therefore promotes a type 1 response and Th1 differentiation. IFN-α, a cytokine produced by virally infected cells early in infection, induces IL-12 and can also switch cells from a Th2 to a Th1 profile. By contrast, early production of the type 2 cytokine IL-4 favors the generation of Th2 cells. NK T cells, M2 macrophages, type 2 innate lymphoid cells (ILC2s), and basophils have all been suggested to be early producers of IL-4.

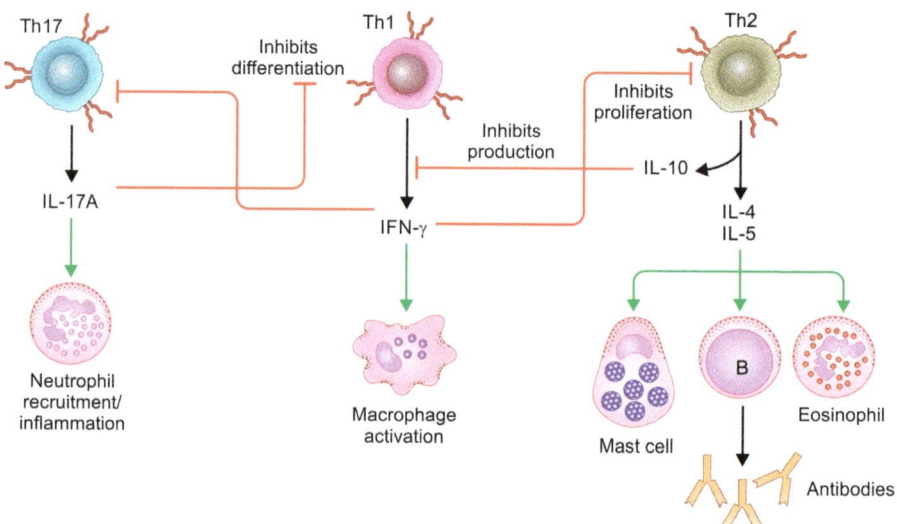

FIG. 9: Selection of effector mechanisms by Th1 and Th2 cells. The cytokine patterns of Th1, Th2, and Th17 cells drive different effector pathways. Th1 cells activate macrophages and are involved in antiviral and inflammatory responses. Th2 cells are involved in humoral responses and allergy. Th17 cells are an important defense at mucosal barriers, recruiting neutrophils to sites of infection and tightening epithelial barriers. Note that certain cytokines, secreted by the cells inhibit other cell lines.

Cytokines from the various Th subsets can **cross-regulate** each other's development, thus:
- IFN-γ secreted by Th1 cells can <u>inhibit</u> the responsiveness of **Th2 cells**.
- The type 3 cytokine *IL-17A* can <u>inhibit</u> the development of *Th1* responses (**Fig. 9**).
- **IL-10** produced by Th2 cells <u>reduces</u> B7 and IL-12 expression by APCs, which in turn inhibits **Th1** activation.

The Th subset balance is affected by levels of expression of cytokines, such as IL-12 or IL-4 but also by expression of cytokine receptors. As an example the high-affinity IL-12R is composed of two chains, β1 and β2, with both chains being constitutively expressed on Th1 cells. Th1, Th2, and Th17 cells express the β1 chain, but expression of the β2 chain is induced by IFN-γ and inhibited by IL-4. Therefore, cytokines reinforce the lineage decisions of the various Th subsets at least in part by controlling the expression of lineage-specific receptors.

What Determines the Type of Immune Response?

The Th cell subsets determine the type of immune response.
- Local patterns of cytokine and hormone expression help to select lymphocyte effector mechanism
- The polarized responses of CD4+ Th cells are based on their profile of cytokine secretion.

Type 1 cytokines including IFN-γ and IL-12, and their actions include:
- Macrophage activation
- Antibody-dependent cell-mediated cytotoxicity
- Delayed-type hypersensitivity

Th2 clones are typified by production of the type 2 cytokines IL-4, IL-5, IL-9, IL-10, and IL-13 (**Fig. 8**). These cells help the humoral immune by:
- IgG1 and IgE isotype switching
- Mucosal immunity

- Stimulation of mast cells, eosinophil growth, and differentiation
- IgA synthesis

Type 3 cytokines produced by Th17 cells include IL-17A, IL-17F, TNF-α, and IL-22. Since many stromal cells express receptors for these cytokines, the effects of Th17 cells can promote inflammation. In addition:
- IL-17A has been proposed to be important for the recruitment of neutrophils and induction of antimicrobial peptides from resident cells.
- IL-17A is important for host defense against *Klebsiella pneumoniae* and *Candida albicans*.

CD8+ T Cells

CD8+ T cells can also be divided into subsets on the basis of cytokine expression.

Most CD8+ CTLs secrete type 1 cytokines and are termed CTL1 cells. CD8+ T cells that stimulate type 2 cytokines are associated with regulatory functions and CD8+ T cells that secrete IL-17A have also been observed. The differentiation of these cells is dictated by CD4+ cell cytokine profile (**Fig. 6**). Thus to summarize:
- IFN-γ and IL-12 may encourage CTL1 generation.
- IL-4 may encourage CTL2 generation.

However, both CTL1 and CTL2 cells can be cytotoxic and kill mainly by a Ca^{2+}/perforin-dependent mechanism (**Fig. 7**).

CD4+ T Cells Display Plasticity between Th1, Th2, and Th17

Studies of Th cells have revealed considerable developmental plasticity. For example, Th17 cells can be induced to produce IFN-γ (a type 1 cytokine) and thereafter shut down production of IL-17A in the presence of IL-12 (**Fig. 10**). Similarly, Th2 cells can be driven to a mixed Th2/1 phenotype, in which cells coexpress IL-4 and IFN-γ, by culture with type I IFNs and IL-12. It is thought that this plasticity may enable rapid site-specific immune responses to infections to occur.

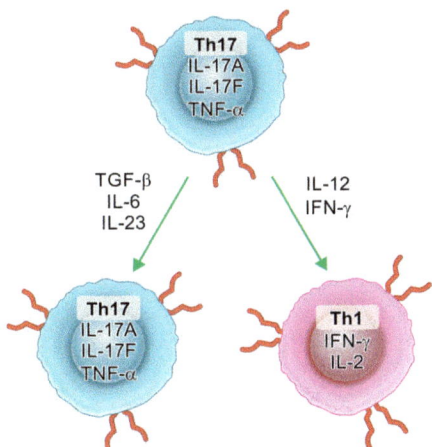

(IFN-γ: interferon gamma; IL: interleukin; TGF-β: transforming growth factor beta; TNF-α: tumor necrosis factor alpha)

FIG. 10: Th17 cells exhibit plasticity in Th1 cytokine environments. Th17 cells can differentiate into Th1 cells in response to IL-12 and interferon gamma (IFN-γ) signaling.

Innate Lymphoid Cells Polarize the Immune Response by Producing Cytokines

The three types of immune response and their characteristic cytokines were originally described in the context of T-helper cells. However, recently, a new family of lymphocytes, called the ILCs (innate lymphoid cells), has been discovered. ILCs are the cells of the lymphoid lineage but, unlike T and B cells, they lack highly variable antigen receptors generated by somatic recombination. They play key roles in innate immunity, tissue repair, and homeostasis at barrier surfaces, including the skin, airways, and gastrointestinal tract.

There are now considered to be **five groups of ILCs, four** of which can be thought of as innate counterparts to T cells (**Fig. 11**):

1. NK cells are the innate counterparts of cytotoxic T cells. Their main function is cytotoxicity, but they also produce the type 1 cytokine IFN-γ.
2. ILC1 are innate counterparts of Th1 cells. They produce IFN-γ, TNF-α, and GM-CSF in response to IL-12 and IL-15.
3. ILC2 are innate counterparts of Th2 cells. They produce IL-4, IL-5, IL-9, and IL-13 in response to IL-25, IL-33, and TSLP.
4. ILC3 are innate counterparts of Th17 cells. They produce IL-22 and IL-17 in response to IL-1β and IL-23.

The fifth group of ILCs is the lymphoid tissue inducer cells (LTis). These were originally considered to be a subset of ILC3 but are now thought of as a separate lineage. They have an important role in the formation of lymph nodes and Peyer's patches. A subset of ILC that produces IL-10 in response to TGF-β has been described, and it is possible that these are innate counterparts to Tregs. However, the development and function of this subset of ILCs is not yet well understood.

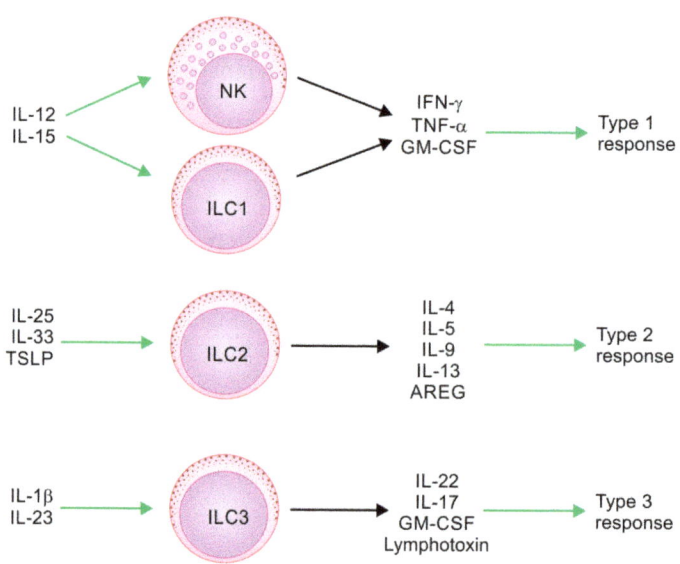

(AREG: amphiregulin; GM-CSF: granulocyte-macrophage colony-stimulating factor; IFN-γ: interferon gamma; IL: interleukin; ILC: innate lymphoid cell; TNF-α: tumor necrosis factor alpha; TSLP: thymic stromal lymphopoietin)

FIG. 11: A depiction of the different types of innate lymphoid cells and their function. IL-12 and IL-15 promote the activity of NK cells and ILC1, both of which produce type 1 cytokines, particularly IFN-γ. IL-25, IL-33, and thymic stromal lymphopoietin (TSLP) promote ILC2 production of type 2 cytokines, including IL-4 and IL-13 as well as amphiregulin (AREG), which promotes epithelial cell growth during wound healing. IL-1β and IL-23 promote ILC3 activity and the production of type 3 cytokines, including IL-22 and IL-17.

Because ILCs respond earlier than T cells, it is likely that they have a critical role in polarizing the immune response, with the cytokines that they produce stimulating the T cells as the adaptive response develops. It has also been argued that, since ILCs are generally tissue-resident and present earlier in development than T cells, they may have a role in initiating the characteristic cytokine milieus of the various tissues.

Immune Regulation and Role of Chemokines

The spatial and temporal production of chemokines by different cell types is an important mechanism of immune regulation. There is good evidence to suggest that the recruitment of Th1, Th2, and Th17 cells is differentially controlled, thereby ensuring the maintenance of locally polarized immune responses.

The expression of different **chemokine** receptors on Th1 cells (CXCR3 and CCR5), Th2 cells (CCR3, CCR4, CCR8), and Th17 (CCR6) allows chemotactic signals to produce the differential localization of T-cell subsets to sites of inflammation.

Chemokines can be induced by cytokines released at sites of inflammation, providing a mechanism for local reinforcement of particular types of response (**Fig. 12**). Once a response is established, the T cells can induce further migration of appropriate effector cells. This is clearly illustrated in type 1 responses where the secondary production of CCL2, CCL3, CXCL10, and CCL5 attracts mononuclear phagocytes to the area of inflammation. Production of IL-17A can drive the expression of CCL20, the ligand for CCR6, recruiting more Th17 cells to the site of inflammation. The ability of cytokines such as TGF-β, IL-12, and IL-4 to influence chemokine or chemokine receptor expression provides a further level of control on cell migration or recruitment.

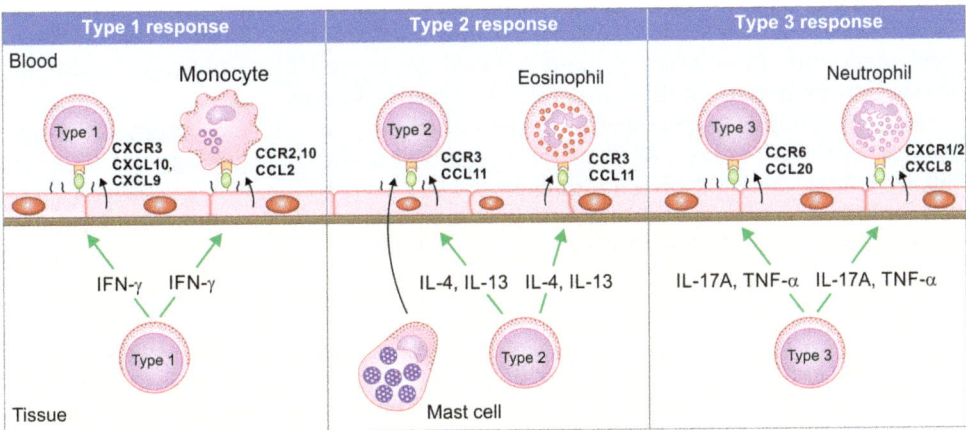

(IFN-γ: interferon gamma; IL: interleukin; TNF-α: tumor necrosis factor alpha)

FIG. 12: Diagram depicting the role of the various chemokines that mediate the 3 type of immune responses. Activated Th1 cells release IFN-γ, which induces chemokines CXCL10 (IP10) and CXCL9. These act on the chemokine receptors CXCR3, which are selectively expressed on Th1 cells, thereby reinforcing this type of response. Macrophage chemotactic protein-1 (MCP-1, CCL2), which attracts macrophages and monocytes, is also induced by IFN-γ. Mast cells release CCL11 (eotaxin) when activated and certain affected tissues like endothelial cells and bronchial epithelium also synthesize this chemokine in response to IL-4 and IL-13 from Th2 cells. Eotaxin acts on CCR3, which is selectively expressed on Th2 cells, thereby reinforcing the Th2 response. Eosinophils and basophils, which mediate allergic responses in airways, also express CCR3. Th17 cells express the chemokine receptor CCR6. IL-17A production by Th17 cells induces expression of CCL20, which acts on CCR6, thus recruiting Th17 cells to the site of infection. Chemokines can therefore potentiate both the initiation and effector phases of a specific type of immune response.

T follicular helper cells express the B-cell follicle homing receptor CXCR5, which allows them to regulate B-cell germinal center formation. Tfh cells express CD40L and secrete IL-21, which mediates the selection and survival of B cells as they undergo proliferation and antibody diversification. Immune responses do not normally occur at certain sites in the body, such as the anterior chamber of the eye and the testes which are referred to as immune privileged sites. The failure to evoke immune responses in these sites is partly because of the presence of inhibitory cytokines, such as TGF-β and IL-10, which inhibit inflammatory responses. The presence of migration inhibition factor (MIF) in the anterior chamber of the eye also inhibits NK-cell activity.

Regulatory T Cells

Although T cells modulate the immune response they can also downregulate immune responses and the most important cell that plays this role is the Treg cells. A naturally occurring population of CD4+ CD25+ Tregs is generated in the thymus. Additionally, CD4+ Tregs can be induced from non-Tregs in the periphery.

Regulatory T cells maintain peripheral tolerance and have important roles in the prevention of autoimmune diseases apart from limiting the levels of immunopathology during an active immune response. Conversely, they are a potential barrier to effective immune surveillance in cancer.

Regulatory T Cell Differentiation is Induced by Foxp3

The immunosuppressive functions of CD4+ cells was initially observed by adoptively transferring T cells depleted of CD25+ cells into immunodeficient mice. This resulted in multiorgan autoimmunity, suggesting that CD25+ cells play an important role in preventing self-reactivity. When the CD25+ T cells were replaced, autoimmune disease was prevented.

Comparison of CD4+ CD25+ Tregs with naive and activated CD4+ T cells shows that Tregs selectively express Foxp3. Mutations in the *Foxp3* gene cause immune dysregulation, polyendocrinopathy enteropathy, and X-linked syndrome (IPEX). Individuals with this disease have increased autoimmune and inflammatory diseases.

A two-stage model for Treg development within the thymus has been proposed. Strongly self-reactive CD4+ T cells upregulate CD25 in response to strong and persistent TCR signals. This then allows for IL-2-driven induction of Foxp3 expression, which represses T-cell IL-2 and IFN-γ expression and imparts the suppressive Treg phenotype. Interestingly, differences in human leukocyte antigen (HLA) alleles have been suggested to affect risk of autoimmunity. For instance, HLA polymorphism can alter the relative abundance of self-epitope-specific Treg cells that can lead to protection or increased risk of autoimmunity.

CD4+ CD25+ Foxp3+ Tregs constitute 5–10% of peripheral CD4+ T cells in both mice and humans and although athymic mice have severely reduced levels of Tregs, it is clear that Foxp3+ Tregs can arise in the periphery. These so-called peripheral (p) Tregs have been extensively studied in vitro. If naive CD4+ T cells are stimulated in the presence of TGF-β, then many cells start expressing Foxp3. The additional presence of retinoic acid is thought to accentuate the conversion of naive CD4+ T cells into Foxp3+ Tregs.

There is a Reciprocal Developmental Relationship between Induced Tregs and Th17 Cells

Induced Treg and Th17 cells are dependent on TGF-β for their development. Thus in the presence of TGF-β, naive CD4+ T cells upregulate Foxp3 and develop into induced Tregs. If there is an addition inflammatory cytokines such as IL-6 or IL-1β, naive T cells develop into inflammatory Th17 cells that secrete cytokines, such as IL-17A, IL-17F, and TNF-α. This dichotomous relationship implies an important role for cytokines derived from the

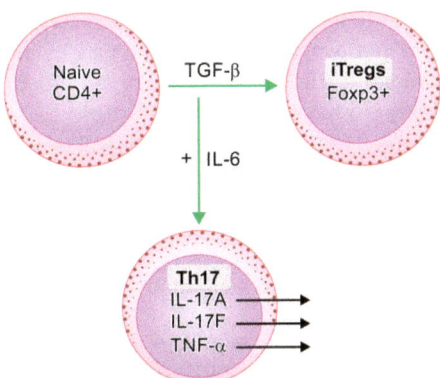

(IL: interleukin; TGF-β: transforming growth factor beta; TNF-α: tumor necrosis factor alpha)

FIG. 13: Reciprocal development of Th17 cells and Tregs is regulated by cyokines. In the presence of TGF-β, naive T cells express Foxp3. However, the presence of IL-6 in combination with TGF-β can drive the differentiation of Th17 cells.

innate immune system in determining the outcome of an adaptive immune response (**Fig. 13**). Such induced Tregs have been seen to arise following allograft transplantation and also after oral administration of antigen. They are also thought to play important roles at mucosal surfaces within the gut. Studies of induced Treg have proven difficult because of a lack of methods to track new Foxp3 expressers during peripheral immune responses.

Regulatory T Cells Suppress the Immune Response using Multiple Mechanisms

Many mechanisms of Treg suppression have been proposed. These include suppression of soluble factors while these have been analyzed in vitro, wherein there is no need for regulatory T-cell populations to home to different locations in order to interact with target cells.

Regulatory T Cells Prevent Immune-mediated Pathology in Infection but can also Dampen Protective T-cell Responses

Although CD4+ Tregs play a vital role in the prevention of autoimmune diseases, their role in infections is less clear. CD4+ Tregs have a protective role against immune-mediated pathology and their ability to suppress is important in reducing inflammation. For example, lesions in the eye in stromal keratitis are less severe in the presence of CD4+ CD25+ Tregs. Also in erythema nodosum leprosum (ENL) reactions Tregs control the reactional changes and suppress inflammation.

CD4+ Tregs can also suppress virus-specific responses. Thus in case of infections, there is enhanced levels of IL-10 and TGF-β, which promote the induction of CD4+ CD25+ Tregs. In chronic viral infections, including HIV, cytomegalovirus (CMV), and herpes simplex virus (HSV) infections, increased numbers of Tregs are responsible for decreased antigen-specific responses by CD4+ and CD8+ T cells, which can lead to disease development.

■ WHERE DO JAKS COME INTO THE PICTURE?

While the overview of the immune response shows that a complex and counterbalance of varied immune cells maintains the homeostasis of the body, the loss of the balance precludes to an autoimmune process. More relevant is the fact that cytokines perpetuate varied cell lines and responses. Cytokines tend to work via signaling pathways and one of the signaling pathway happens to be the JAK-STAT pathway. While not all cytokines mediate their action via the JAK-STAT pathway, all type 1 and type 2 cytokines have JAK-STAT as an intermediary signaling molecule. Thus as a corollary, any disorder with a predominant cytokine basis of this pathway is a target for JAKinibs drugs.

In the following chapters (see Chapters 2 and 3), we will examine the signaling pathway of cytokines, how to suppress them, and the role of JAKinibs drugs.

■ REFERENCES

1. Leonard WJ, Lin JX. Strategies to therapeutically modulate cytokine action. Nat Rev Drug Discov. 2023;22(10):827-54.
2. Moutsopoulos HM, Zampeli E. (2020). Immunology and Rheumatology in Questions. [online] Available from https://doi.org/10.1007/978-3-030-56670-8_1 [Last accessed December, 2023].
3. Roitt I, Brostoff J, Male D, Roth D, Male V. Regulation of The Immune Response. Immunology E-Book, 9th edition. Elsevier: OHCE; 2020. https://bookshelf.health.elsevier.com/books/9780702078477
4. Abbas AK, Lichtman AH, Pillai S (Eds). Cellular and Molecular Immunology, 10th edition. South Asia Edition, E-Book. Elsevier Health Sciences; 2021.

CHAPTER 2

Cytokines Signaling Pathway and Role of JAK-STAT Pathway

Kabir Sardana

"The person who does not read has no advantage over the person who cannot read."
—Mark Twain

Overview

- Introduction
- Cytokines and the Signaling Pathways
- JAK-STAT Pathway
- Therapeutic and Experimental Inhibitions of Cytokines

■ INTRODUCTION

The previous chapter discussed the immunology and the role of varied cells and the fact that the cytokines can play a role in cell differentiation and modulation of the activity of the varied cell types. In this chapter, we will highlight the signaling pathways and the role of Janus kinase-signal transducer and activator of transcription (JAK-STAT) receptors.

Autoimmune versus Autoinflammatory Disorders

Autoimmune diseases refer to a spectrum of conditions in which the immune system mistakenly attacks one's own body. This response lead to a dysregulated adaptive immunity (mediated by B and T lymphocytes) toward anatomical self-antigens. There is an association with certain human leukocyte antigen (HLA) genes that are expressed on antigen-presenting cells, which result in presentation of antigens to effector T cells in an interactive process required for antigen-specific T-cell activation. Effector T cells then generate local inflammation by producing inflammatory cytokines or directly damaging the tissues, whereas CD4+CD25+ regulatory T (Treg) cells counteract the inflammatory response to maintain immune homeostasis in tissues. A large number of disorders including vitiligo, alopecia areata, and lichen planus have an autoimmune basis.

Autoinflammatory syndromes are a rare set of disorders caused mostly by genetic mutations that affect <u>innate immune cells</u> (such as macrophages or neutrophils) and lead to uncontrolled activation of the immune system when there is no actual infection. These patients often respond better to select anti-inflammatory drugs [such as anti-tumor necrosis factor (TNF) or anti-interleukin-1 beta (IL-1β)] but not to broad immunosuppressives. Examples of autoinflammatory disorders include familial Mediterranean fever, TNF receptor-associated periodic syndrome, cryopyrin-associated periodic syndromes, deficiency of the IL-1 receptor antagonist (IL-1Rα), deficiency of the IL-36Rα, and interferonopathies.

CYTOKINES AND THE SIGNALING PATHWAYS

Cytokines are secreted glycoproteins that act as intercellular messengers to control the hematopoietic and immune systems and the inflammatory response. The term "cytokine" arises from the Greek κύτος and κίνησις (cell and movement) consistent with their ability to mobilize cells to sites of infection and inflammation. While various families of cytokines have been described, we will focus on the class 1 and class 2 cytokines as their action is mediated by the JAK/STAT cascade.

As shown in **Figure 1**, there are three major shared chains utilized by **Class I cytokines**. These are gp130, beta common and gamma common, utilized by IL-6, IL-3, and IL-2 family cytokines, respectively. In addition to these, there are two other shared chains used by cytokines in the IL-4/13 and IL-12/23 subgroups. Finally, there are the homodimeric receptors, consisting of two identical chains such as those used by erythropoietin (EPO), thrombopoietin (TPO), growth hormone (GH), prolactin (PRL), leptin, and granulocyte colony-stimulating factor (G-CSF). Within each of these classes, the cytokine IL-12Rβ2 receptor stoichiometry and organization can differ. A common theme within the nonhomodimeric receptors is that there will be a cytokine-specific chain (nominally the "alpha" chain) that recognizes cytokine with high affinity, and the resulting dimer will then recruit a "shared" chain in order to initiate signaling.

The **Class II** family cytokines encompass the interferons (IFNs-α, β, γ, λ, ε, κ, ω) and IL-10 family cytokines. Signaling via Class II cytokine receptors (unlike Class I) adheres to a more common set of rules regarding stoichiometry and receptor assembly. Each Class II receptor is a heterodimer and each of these receptors associate with one molecule of cytokine to initiate signaling.

Early induction of the majority of inflammatory transcripts depends on *transcription factor* networks including nuclear factor kappa B (NF-κB) (canonical and noncanonical), STATs, nuclear factor of activated T cells (NFATs), and interferon-regulatory factors (IRFs).

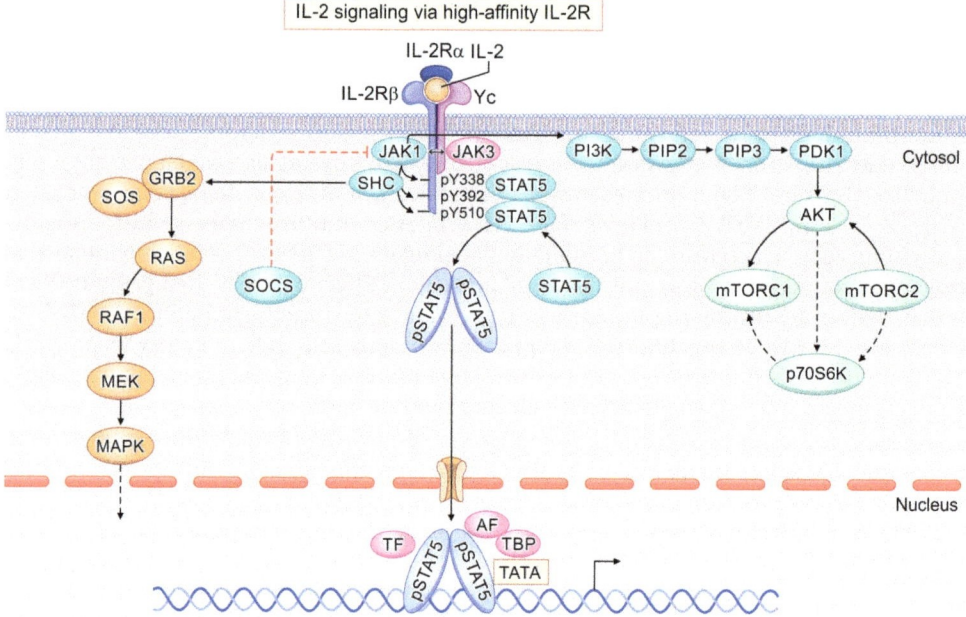

(JAK: janus kinase; STAT: signal transducer and activator of transcription)

FIG. 1: Depiction of the salient cytokine signaling pathways using interleukin (IL-2) as an example.

However, the net production of the corresponding proteins depends, in part, on mitogen-activated protein kinases (MAPK) and molecular programs that regulate transcript stability and translation.

Thus, following ligand binding and receptor dimerization, **three** major signaling pathways are activated by cytokines: JAK-STAT, MAP kinase, and phosphoinositide 3-kinase (PI3K)–Akt (**Fig. 1**). Notably, MAPK and PI3K are activated by a range of signals beyond cytokines.

■ JAK-STAT PATHWAY

The JAK-STAT signaling pathway is an elegantly simple signaling cascade in which the cytokine requires only three components (receptor, kinase, and transcription factor) to elicit a response. JAK-STAT is largely restricted to type I and type II cytokines.

Each *JAK* consists of four distinct domains: An N-terminal FERM domain followed by an SH2 domain and two kinase domains. JAKs have both catalytic and pseudo-kinase domains (originally designated as JAK homology domains 1 and 2, with the catalytically active kinase domain at the C terminus). The four domains can be further divided into seven partitions referred to as JH1–7. JH1 and JH2 are located at the C-terminal end of the protein, and JH3–7 is located at the N-terminal end. These nonreceptor tyrosine kinases interact with the cytoplasmic domains of type I and type II cytokine receptors (**Fig. 2**).

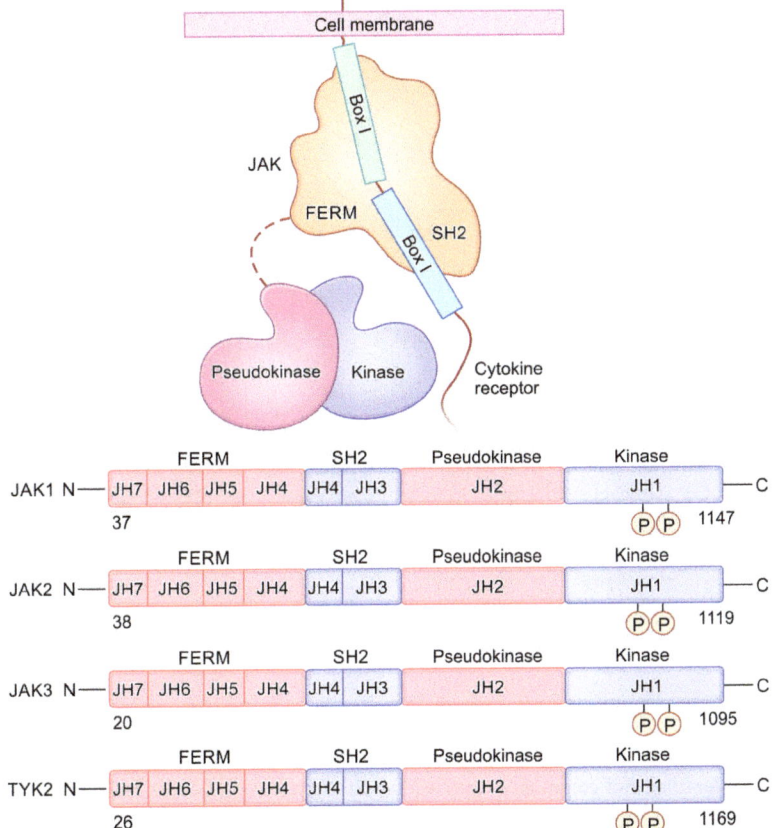

FIG. 2: A depictive diagram that shows the components of the JAK receptor. The diagram below shows the components of the various JAK subtypes.

There are **four JAKs**—JAK1, JAK2, JAK3, and TYK2. **JAK3** is *inducible,* whereas the others are constitutive. JAK3 acts in combination with JAK1 and is activated by γc-family cytokines (**Fig. 3**). JAK2 is the JAK that is used by all cytokines that use receptor homodimers. Thus not all possible JAK pairs are used, suggesting that some would pair better or certain pairs have simply not arisen during evolution. Thus, some combinations of JAKs are physiologically favored, creating new cytokine receptor combinations that pair with distinctive JAKs resulting in novel biological effects. JAKs transduce signaling of IL-2R, IL-4R, IL-5R, IL-6R, IL-13R, and type I IFNs, which all have been validated in different diseases such as rheumatic arthritis (RA), atopic dermatitis, and asthma. TYK2 is activated downstream after receptor binding by IL-23, IL-12, and type I IFNs and has a prominent role in psoriasis (**Fig. 3**).

After the JAKs are activated the **STAT proteins** are activated (**Fig. 4**). The STATs are a family of proteins named for their dual roles of (1) transducing signals from cytokines and (2) promoting transcription of specific genes. The STATs predominantly reside in the cytoplasm as inactive dimers but are rapidly activated upon initiation of cytokine signaling and translocate into the nucleus. There are <u>seven</u> mammalian STATs (STAT1–4, STAT5a, STAT5b, and STAT6). After phosphorylation, STAT proteins can form either homodimers or heterodimers based on the interaction of the STAT SH2 domain, located between the DNA

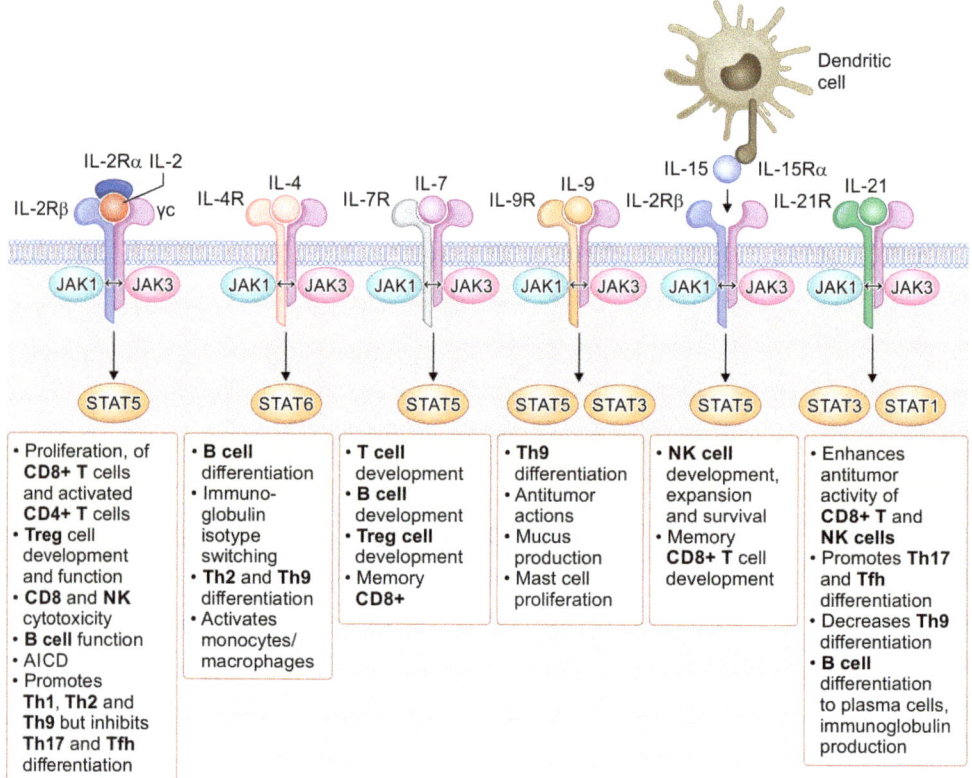

(IL: interleukin; JAK: janus kinase; NK: natural killer; STAT: signal transducer and activator of transcription)

FIG. 3: The cellular effects of common γ-chain (γc) family of cytokines. IL-2, IL-4, IL-7, IL-9, IL-15, and IL-21, which activate JAK1 and JAK3, with JAK3 binding to γc. For each cytokine, specific STAT proteins are activated and lead to varied immune effects.

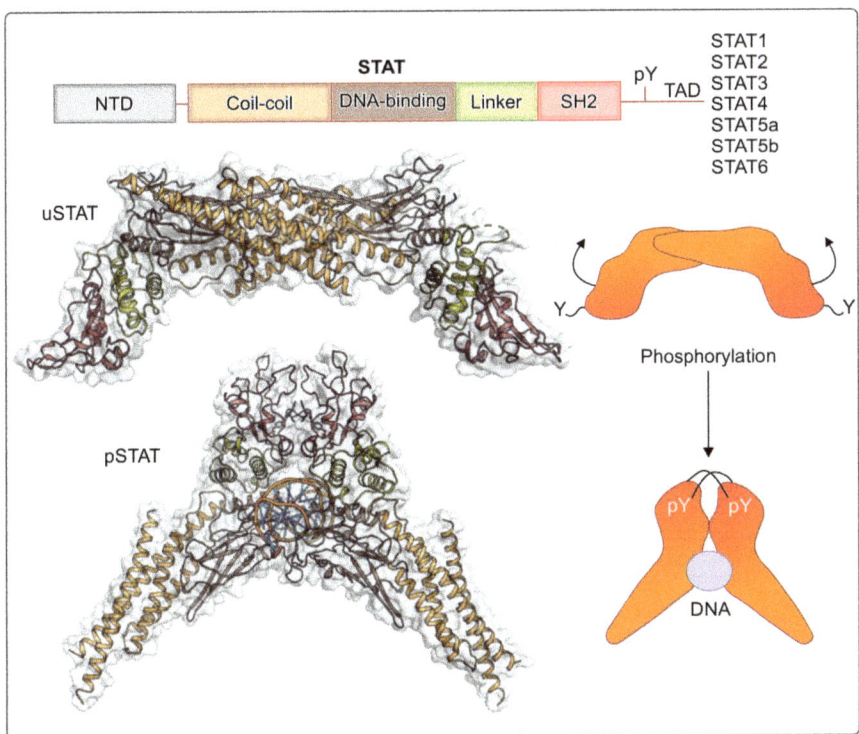

FIG. 4: The signal transducers and activators of transcription (STATs) are a family of latent transcription factors that are activated by phosphorylation following cytokine exposure. Unphosphorylated STAT (uSTAT) exists as an antiparallel dimer in the cytoplasm (upper). The SH2 domain (red) of uSTAT binds to phosphotyrosines in cytokine receptors, which allows JAK to phosphorylate a specific tyrosine located between the SH2 and transactivation domain (TAD). This phosphotyrosine is then targeted by the SH2 domain of the other monomer inducing a large rotation between the two subunits of the dimer and allowing phosphorylated STAT (pSTAT) to occupy its DNA-binding competent dimeric structure (lower).

binding domain and the C-terminal tyrosine, with the C-terminal pTyr on the partner STAT and vice versa, thereby creating bivalent interactions. After nuclear translocation, STAT dimers bind to specific DNA motifs.

Many regulators **inhibit** the activation of the JAK-STAT signaling pathway. There are **three main types** of JAK-STAT regulators: Suppressors of cytokine signaling (SOCS), protein inhibitors of activated STATs (PIASs), and protein tyrosine phosphatases.

To understand the role of the varied JAK inhibitor drugs, it is useful to know the interaction of cytokines families and JAK/STAT as given in the **Table 1** and this can be used to predict the action of the JAK inhibitor drugs in varied disorders, which is possible if the tissue cytokine data in the disorders is available.

As the differentiation and further cytokine secretion of varied subtypes of CD4 cells are determined by cytokines their action is also mediated by JAK/STAT pathway (**Fig. 5**).

Thereby, JAK-STAT-dependent signaling is involved in many fundamental biological processes, including apoptosis, proliferation, migration, development, and differentiation of a variety of cell types present in all organs of the body. Inhibition of one or more JAKs or STATs can lead to the inhibition of other family members. Not all the actions of type I/II cytokines in various tissues have been clarified, and thus the molecular consequences/effects of JAK/STAT inhibition are currently not fully understood.[1]

TABLE 1 Families of interleukin transduction signals via the JAK/STAT pathway.

Classification	Cytokines	JAKs	STATs
Class I cytokines signaling			
IL-2 family	IL-2, IL-4, IL-7, IL-9, IL-15, IL-21	JAK1, JAK3	STAT1, STAT3, STAT5, STAT6
	IL-4, IL-13	JAK1, TYK2	STAT6
IL-3 family	IL-3, IL-5, GM-CSF	JAK2	STAT5
IL-6 family	IL-6, IL-11, IL-31, LIF, CNTF, CT1, CLC, OSM	JAK1, TYK2, JAK2	STAT1, STAT3, STAT6
IL-12/23	IL-12, IL-23	TYK2/JAK2	STAT3, STAT4
Homodimeric (tall)	LEP	JAK2	STAT5
	G-CSF	JAK1*	STAT3
Homodimeric (short)	TPO, EPO, GH, PRL	JAK2	STAT5
Class II cytokine signaling			
Type I IFN	IFN-α, IFN-β, IFN-E, IFN-κ	JAK1, TYK2	STAT1, STAT2
Type II IFN	IFN-γ	JAK1, JAK2	STAT1, STAT3, STAT5
Type III IFN	IFN-γ1 (IL-29), IFN-γ2 (IL-28A), IFN-γ3 (IL-28B)	TYK2, JAK1	STAT1, STAT2
IL-10 family	IL-10, IL-19, IL-20, IL-22, IL-24, IL-26	TYK2, JAK1	STAT1, STAT3, STAT5

*JAK1 predominance with assistance of JAK2 and TYK2.

(CNTF: ciliary neurotrophic growth Factor; CT1: cardiotrophin 1; CLC: cardiotrophin-like cytokine; OSM: oncostatin M; EPO: erythropoietin; GH: growth hormone; GM-CSF: granulocyte monophosphate colony-stimulating factor; IL: interleukin; IFN: interferon; JAK/STAT: Janus kinase-signal transducer and activator of transcription; PRL: prolactin; TPO: thrombopoietin)

JAK-STAT Pathway and Diseases

There is emerging evidence that JAK-STAT activation can play dual roles in diseases. Hyperactivation of the JAK-STAT pathway has been implicated in the poor outcomes of many diseases including melanomas, glioblastomas, and head, neck, lung, pancreatic, breast, rectal, and prostate cancers. Also mutations and polymorphisms can lead to autoimmune diseases and immune-mediated cancers (**Fig. 6**). Conversely, favorable regulatory roles of the JAK-STAT pathway have been demonstrated in head and neck squamous cell carcinomas and prostate and colorectal cancers.

What determines cytokine specificity?

With only four JAKs and seven STAT proteins but a myriad of cytokines, it is evident that JAKs and STATs by themselves cannot fully determine specificity, but they contribute to it. Some cytokines activate more than one STAT, but often one is dominantly activated. Different STATs can exert competing actions (e.g., STAT1 vs. STAT3, STAT3 vs. STAT5, and so forth), and this in part explains why different cytokines exert different effects. An added complexity is STAT dimerization versus tetramerization. Moreover, full activation of some STAT proteins requires serine phosphorylation. Although the original dogma was that unphosphorylated STATs are in the cytosol and undergo nuclear translocation only after tyrosine phosphorylation, some unphosphorylated STATs (e.g., STAT1, STAT2, STAT3, and STAT5A) are in the nucleus. Besides STAT activation, MAPK and PI3K–Akt can

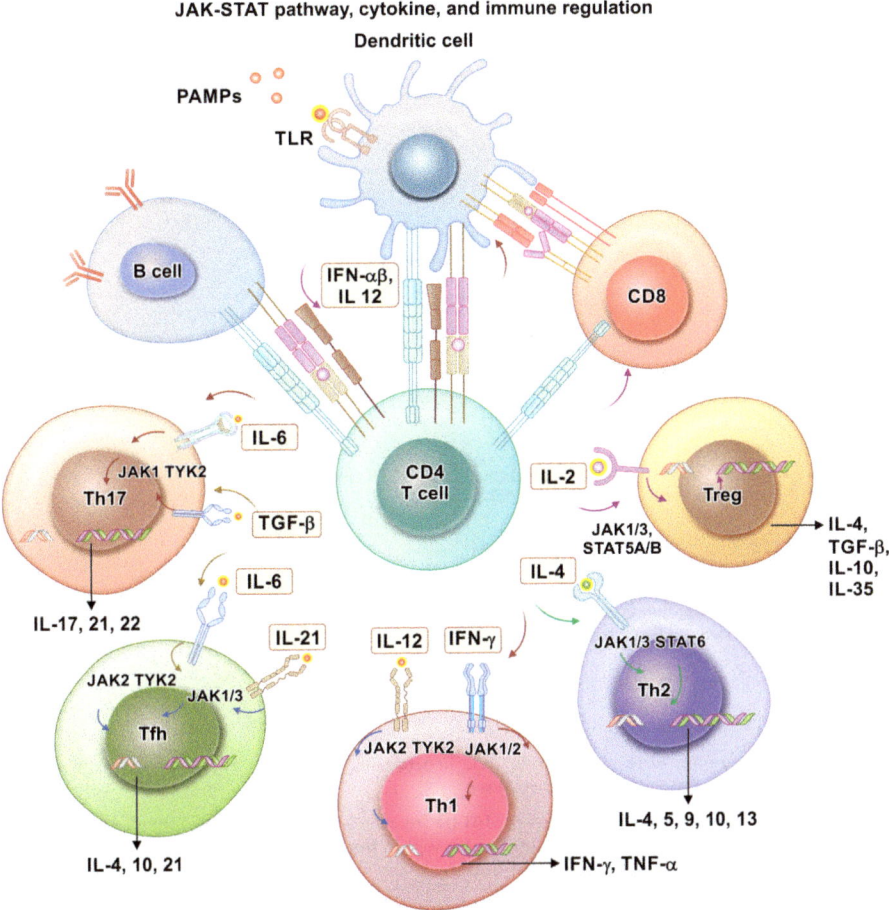

(IFN: interferon; IL: interleukin; JAK: janus kinase; STAT: signal transducer and activator of transcription; TGF: transforming growth factor; TLR: toll-like receptor)

FIG. 5: A depiction of the role of JAK pathway in the differentiation of CD4 T cells. IFN gamma and IL-12 determine Th1 cell differentiation via JAK1/2 TYK2 and STAT1 and STAT4 . IL-4 upregulates via JAK1/3 and STAT6 to activates Th2 cell differentiation. IL-6 and TGF-β determines Th17 cell differentiation via STAT3. IL-6 and IL-12 mediate T follicular helper cell differentiation via STAT3. IL-2 induces Treg cell differentiation.

be activated by cytokine signals. Although STAT activation contributes to gene regulation and differentiation, MAPK to proliferation and PI3K–Akt to cell survival, each pathway can have multiple effects, and the relative potency of activation of each signaling pathway presumably determines or influences the net signal transduced into the cell.

Negative Regulation of Cytokine Signaling

Negative regulation of cytokine signaling is essential; otherwise, a stimulus could lead to uncontrolled growth or autoimmunity. Negative regulation can occur at many steps, including at the level of transcription, translation, posttranslational modification, and protein stability.

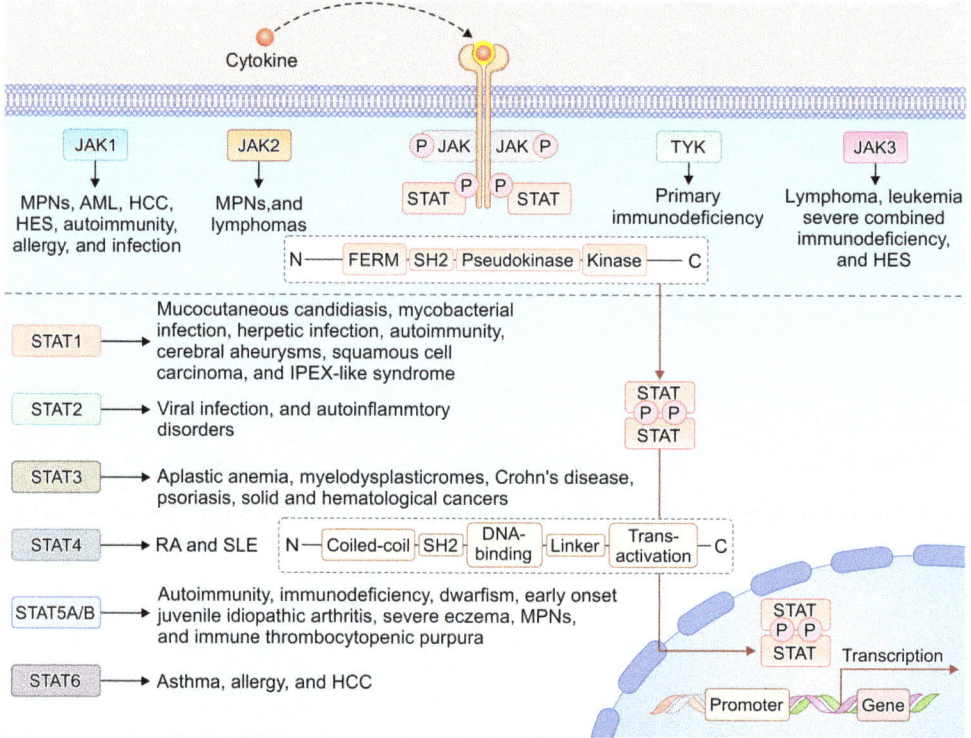

(AML: acute myeloid leukemia; MPN: myelofibrosis; HCC: hepatocellular carcinoma; HES: hypereosinophilic syndrome; RA: rheumatoid arthritis; SLE: systemic lupus erythematosus)

FIG. 6: A depiction of the mutations of the JAK-STAT pathway in human disease and the diseases they cause. The most frequent site of disease-causing mutations is within the SH2 domain in both JAKs and STATs.

■ THERAPEUTIC AND EXPERIMENTAL INHIBITIONS OF CYTOKINES

The drugs that can target the JAK/STAT pathway can be classified into three broad types (**Fig. 7**).
1. Cytokine or receptor antibodies
2. JAK inhibitors
3. STAT inhibitors (**Fig. 7**)

Monoclonal Antibodies

Although understanding signaling pathways in inflammatory and autoimmune diseases is challenging, preclinical and clinical research has been greatly instructive for therapeutic development. Biologics (such as antibody antagonists or fusion proteins) have validated several pathogenic pathways involved in these diseases. Thus, there are a wide array of drugs that target cytokine receptors and/or ligands (such as TNF and IL-1), leading to cellular depletion and reduction of pathogenic cellular response (such as anti-CD20 antibodies for B-cell depletion to limit autoantibody production or B cell-mediated antigen-presenting cell function) or inhibition of cellular differentiation [such as inhibition of macrophage colony-stimulating factor 1 receptor (CSF1R) to reduce macrophage differentiation].

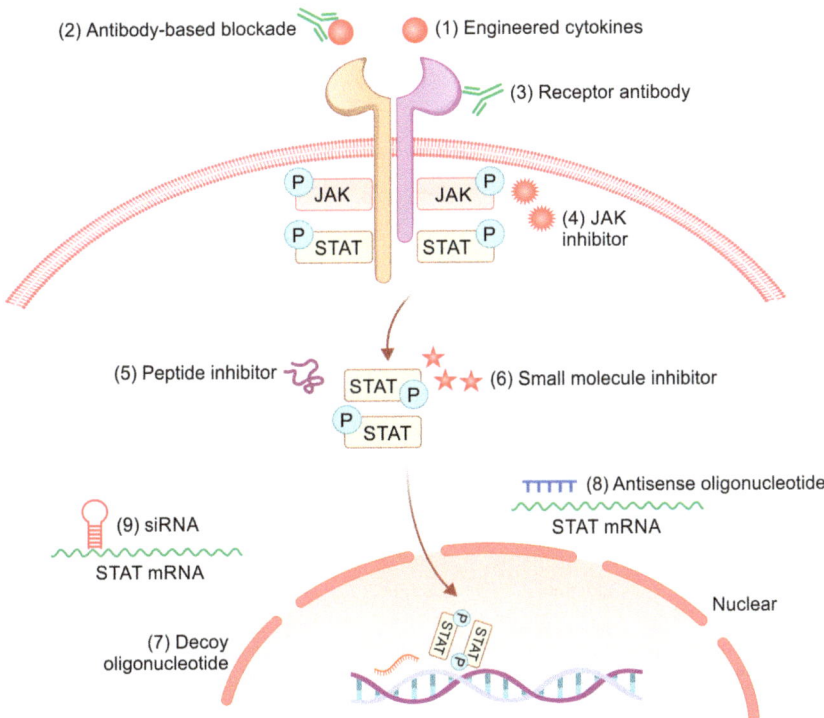

(JAK: janus kinase; STAT: signal transducer and activator of transcription)

FIG. 7: A diagram that shows the various steps and agents that can block the JAK STAT pathway.

Collectively, antibodies to a broad range of type I and II cytokines and their receptors, including interferon-alpha receptor 1 (IFNAR1), IFN-γ, IL-2Rα, IL-4Rα, IL-5, IL-5Rα, IL-6, IL-6R, IL-12/IL-23 p40, IL-13, IL-23 p19, and thymic stromal lymphopoietin (TSLP) have been approved for therapeutic use, as well as TNF, TNF receptor, IL-1-based antibodies, IL-17/IL-17R, and others [e.g., vascular endothelial growth factor (VEGF), transforming growth factor (**Fig. 8**).

Engineered Cytokines

This category includes recombinant IL-2 approved for the treatment of metastatic melanoma and renal cell carcinoma; type 1 IFNs are used for the treatment of hepatitis C virus; IFN-α used for treating the viral infections, and TNF is a treatment of cancer. Cytokine–antibody fusions are novel biopharmaceuticals that increase the therapeutic index of cytokine "payloads."

Inhibiting JAKs and STATs

Kinases (518 encoded in genome) are the enzymes that phosphorylate up to one-third of the proteome, and drugs targeting them are of use in cancer, inflammatory, and neurodegenerative diseases.[2] Owing to the distribution of select kinases in multiple signaling cascades in immune cells, the use of small-molecule kinase inhibitors have the potential to inhibit inflammation in a targeted fashion. Emerging data suggest that *combination therapy* with nonoverlapping therapeutics (such as combinations of biologics

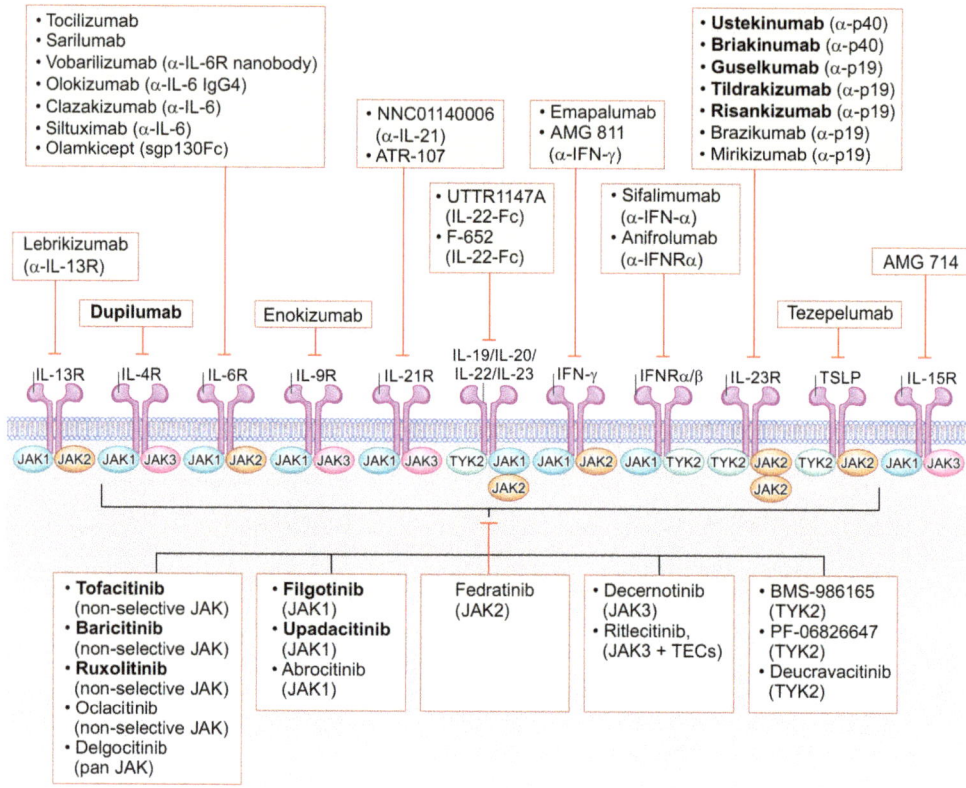

(IFN: interferon; IL: interleukin; JAK: janus kinase; TSLP: thymic stromal lymphopoietin)

FIG. 8: Overview of biologicals and JAK inhibitor that inhibit cytokines. As is obvious JAK inhibitor have a pan cytokine suppressive potential.

and kinase inhibitors) may be more effective than single agents.[3] Thus, it is essential for clinicians to understand signaling pathway and the role of kinases and explains their utility in a wide variety of disorders.

STAT Inhibitors

Signal transducer and activator of transcription proteins mediate the actions of cytokines, and selective inhibition of one of the STATs can shift the balance toward another phenotype. Gain-of-function mutations of STAT3 and STAT5B have been reported in patients with hematopoietic and solid malignancies, with many of the mutations affecting the SH2 domain, which results in sustained STAT activation by making the proteins more resistant to dephosphorylation (**Fig. 6**). A range of STAT3 inhibitors have been developed, including small-molecule inhibitors and a cyclic STAT3 decoy oligonucleotide, with STAT5 inhibitors also under evaluation. One of the best-known molecule is STATTIC (STAT three inhibitory compound), and other inhibitors have been identified for STAT3 and have been recently reviewed.[4] In principle, depending on the STAT, specific STAT inhibition may be more specific than JAK inhibition, although this is more relevant to JAK 3, which is only used by six cytokines.

JAK Inhibitors

Inhibiting JAKs has the potential to change the oral therapeutics of many disorders (**Table 2**) and as they tend to inhibit multiple cytokines families of type 1 and type 2 cytokines, they have a rapid effect and would be more effective than biologicals (**Fig. 8**).

Janus kinase inhibitors, both reversible and irreversible, have been advanced to clinical evaluation with varying degrees of selectivity (**Fig. 2**). Covalent inhibitors bind irreversibly to kinase pockets or to the adjacent chemically reactive amino acid (usually cysteine, lysine or aspartic acid) to form a bond and block activity. JAK inhibitors have been developed with a range of efficacy, including for plaque psoriasis, psoriatic arthritis, juvenile arthritis, ankylosing spondyloarthritis, ulcerative colitis, atopic dermatitis, alopecia areata, graft-versus-host disease (GVHD), myeloproliferative neoplasms, vitiligo, and coronavirus disease 2019 (COVID-19).

Tofacitinib was produced as a JAK3-preferring, but only partially selective inhibitor, with weaker effects on JAK1 and JAK2. Tofacitinib inhibits signaling by all six γc-family cytokines

TABLE 2: JAK inhibitors.

Inhibitor	Brand name	Target	Approved for disease	FDA approved
Tofacitinib	Xeljanz	JAK3, JAK1, more weakly JAK2 and TYK2	Rheumatoid arthritis, psoriatic arthritis, juvenile arthritis, ankylosing spondyloarthritis, and ulcerative colitis	2012
Baricitinib	Olumiant	JAK1, JAK2, moderate TYK2	Rheumatoid arthritis, atopic dermatitis, alopecia areata, COVID-19, and vitiligo	2017
Upadacitinib	Rinvoq	JAK1	Rheumatoid arthritis, psoriatic arthritis, ankylosing spondylo-arthritis, ulcerative colitis, and atopic dermatitis	2019
Filgotinib	Jyseleca	JAK1	Rheumatoid arthritis, being evaluated for ulcerative colitis	Approved by EU and Japan
Peficitinib	Smyraf	JAK3	Rheumatoid arthritis	Approved by Japan and Korea but not by the FDA
Abrocitinib	Cibinqo	JAK1	Atopic dermatitis	2022
Delgocitinib	Corectim	JAK1, JAK2, JAK3, TYK2	Atopic dermatitis	2020
Ruxolitinib	Jakafi	JAK1, JAK2, weakly TYK2	Atopic dermatitis, GVHD, myeloproliferative disease	2011
Deucravacitinib	Sotyktu	TYK2	Adults with moderate to severe plaque psoriasis	2022
Fedratinib	Inrebic	JAK2	Myeloproliferative disease	2019
Pacritinib	Vonjo	JAK2	Adults with intermediate- or high-risk primary or secondary myelofibrosis who have platelet levels below 50,000 µL^{-1}	2022

(COVID-19: coronavirus disease 2019; EU: European Union; FDA: Food and Drug Administration; GVHD: graft-versus-host disease; JAK: janus kinase)

(**Figs. 3 and 8**). Originally approved for the treatment of rheumatoid arthritis, tofacitinib now has a range of uses. In **dermatology** apart from tofacitinib, baricitinib (alopecia areata, atopic dermatitis), abrocitinib (atopic dermatitis), delgocitinib (hand-eczema), upadacitinib (atopic dermatitis), deucravacitinib (psoriasis), and recently ritlecitinib (alopecia areata) have been approved for varied indications and an array of novel JAKib drugs are under trial.

It remains unclear whether specific JAK3 inhibitors will be therapeutically superior to JAK inhibitors that inhibit not only JAK3 but also other JAKs. Inhibition of other JAKs could be deleterious (e.g., inhibition of JAK2 could result in defective erythropoiesis given the role of JAK2 in erythropoiesis); however, targeting another JAK to some degree (e.g., JAK1) might enhance the inhibition of γc-family cytokines, all of which use both JAK1 and JAK3. It is also possible that inhibiting more than one JAK could dampen the effects of more than one cytokine, to therapeutic advantage or disadvantage. The rationale of selective versus nonselective JAKib in the efficacy or adverse events is a topic that still needs to be assessed in head to head trials.

■ CONCLUSION

In this chapter, we have discussed the cytokine signaling pathway and focused on the JAK-STAT signaling pathways and also covered the various methods to inhibit cytokines. While biologicals largely inhibit a single cytokine (**Fig. 8**), JAK inhibitors can by their action inhibit multiple cytokines, though the actual in vivo effect depends on the tissue concentration, and thus the clinical effects may be reversible and thus has the advantage of a quick rapid and reversible effect. In the next chapter, we will focus largely on JAK inhibitors as a class of drugs.

■ REFERENCES

1. Bonelli M, Kerschbaumer A, Kastrati K, Ghoreschi K, Gadina M, Heinz LX, et al. Selectivity, efficacy and safety of JAKinibs: new evidence for a still evolving story. Ann Rheum Dis. 2023:ard-2023-223850.
2. Ferguson FM, Gray NS. Kinase inhibitors: the road ahead. Nat Rev Drug Discov. 2018;17:353-77.
3. Boleto G, Kanagaratnam L, Drame M, Salmon JH. Safety of combination therapy with two bDMARDs in patients with rheumatoid arthritis: a systematic review and meta-analysis. Semin Arthritis Rheum. 2018;49:35-42.
4. Hu X, Li J, Fu M, Zhao X, Wang W. The JAK/STAT signaling pathway: from bench to clinic. Signal Transduct. Target Ther. 2021;6:402.

CHAPTER 3

JAK Inhibitors: An Overview

Kabir Sardana

"Common sense is the collection of prejudices acquired by age eighteen."
—Albert Einstein

Overview

- Rationale and Development of Janus Kinase Inhibitors
- Janus Kinase-signal Transducer and Activator of Transcription Pathway, Function, and Classification
- Overview of Salient Janus Kinase Inhibitors in Clinical Practice
- Topical Janus Kinase Inhibitors

■ RATIONALE AND DEVELOPMENT OF JANUS KINASE INHIBITORS

The inhibition of key cytokines by targeting their signal transduction pathways with small molecules was first articulated in 1995 and was based on genetic data which revealed that loss of function leads to diseases. Based on existing data, it was suggested that it is possible to block cytokines by developing highly specific inhibitors of protein kinases, by designing small molecules that could block the adenosine triphosphate (ATP) docking site.

Prior to the widespread use of Janus kinase inhibitors (**JAKinibs**), a large number of biological disease-modifying antirheumatic drugs (**bDMARDs**) had been licensed in the field of rheumatology and many other areas (oncology, dermatology, gastroenterology, and neurology). However, if the existing drugs are analyzed in context of the vast evidence generated from rheumatology literature, it will be obvious (**Fig. 1**) that most of these bDMARDs are efficacious for one or just a few diseases, except for tumor necrosis factor (TNF) inhibitors, which are highly efficacious across all these disorders including inflammatory bowel disease (IBD) and uveitis. This raises certain interesting and difficult to explain conundrums.

(1) Why do so many agents work selectively in one or few disorders, while TNF inhibitors act so widely across diseases and (2) why in rheumatic arthritis (RA) and psoriasis arthritis (PsA), the response rates of all these different targeted therapies are very similar. It has been hypothesized that this may be due to the pivotal role of proinflammatory cytokines, especially TNF-α as TNF-α represents a common shared pathway that is directly or indirectly targeted by drugs with different modes of action across diseases.[1] Consistent

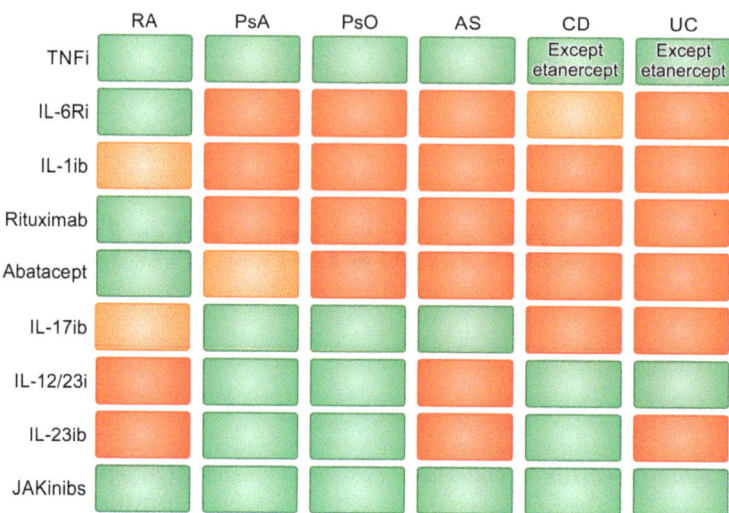

[AS: ankylosing spondylitis; CD: Crohn's disease; i: inhibitor(s); IL: interleukin; JAKinibs: Janus kinase inhibitors; PsA: psoriatic arthritis; PsO: psoriasis; RA: rheumatoid arthritis; TNF: tumor necrosis factor; UC: ulcerative colitis]

FIG. 1: Efficacy of various approved agents across different therapies. [Green: good efficacy; orange: low efficacy (some not approved for the respective indication); red: no efficacy (not approved for the respective indication).

Source: Bonelli M, Kerschbaumer A, Kastrati K, Ghoreschi K, Gadina M, Heinz LX, et al. Selectivity, efficacy and safety of JAKinibs: new evidence for a still evolving story. Ann Rheum Dis. 2023;0:1-22.

with this theory, combinations of bDMARDs do not exhibit increased efficacy, while the increase in serious infections suggests that there is contrary interference with more than one immunological pathway.[2]

Tumor necrosis factor alpha does not signal via JAKs, but uses the nuclear factor kappa B (NF-κB) and mitogen-activated protein kinase (MAPK) pathways. Thus drugs that inhibit the p38 MAPK, NF-κB, and other signaling cascades, such as spleen tyrosine kinase (Syk) used by Fc receptors or Bruton tyrosine kinase (BTK) used by B cell receptors have been a focus of clinical research. But neither p38 nor Syk inhibition showed significant efficacy, while phase II data for BTK inhibition showed some efficacy, but the development for RA was apparently discontinued. It is a riddle why inhibition of other molecules does not work to a similar extent as does JAKinibs.

■ JANUS KINASE-SIGNAL TRANSDUCER AND ACTIVATOR OF TRANSCRIPTION PATHWAY, FUNCTION, AND CLASSIFICATION

Revising the Janus Kinase-signal Transducer and Activator of Transcription Pathway

More than 20 years ago, groundbreaking research from the laboratories of James Darnell, George Stark, and Ian Kerr mainly revealed the molecular specifics of the Janus kinase-signal transducer and activator of transcription (JAK-STAT) pathway. The cytokine needs the receptor, kinase, and transcription factor in an ingeniously straightforward signaling cascade in order to trigger a reaction (**Fig. 2**). Each cytokine binds to a specific receptor on the surface of its target cell, which acts via the JAK-STAT pathway (see Chapter 2). During the classical activation of JAK-STAT, there is an induction of alternative signaling pathways associated with cellular stress, notably the phosphoinositide 3-kinase/protein

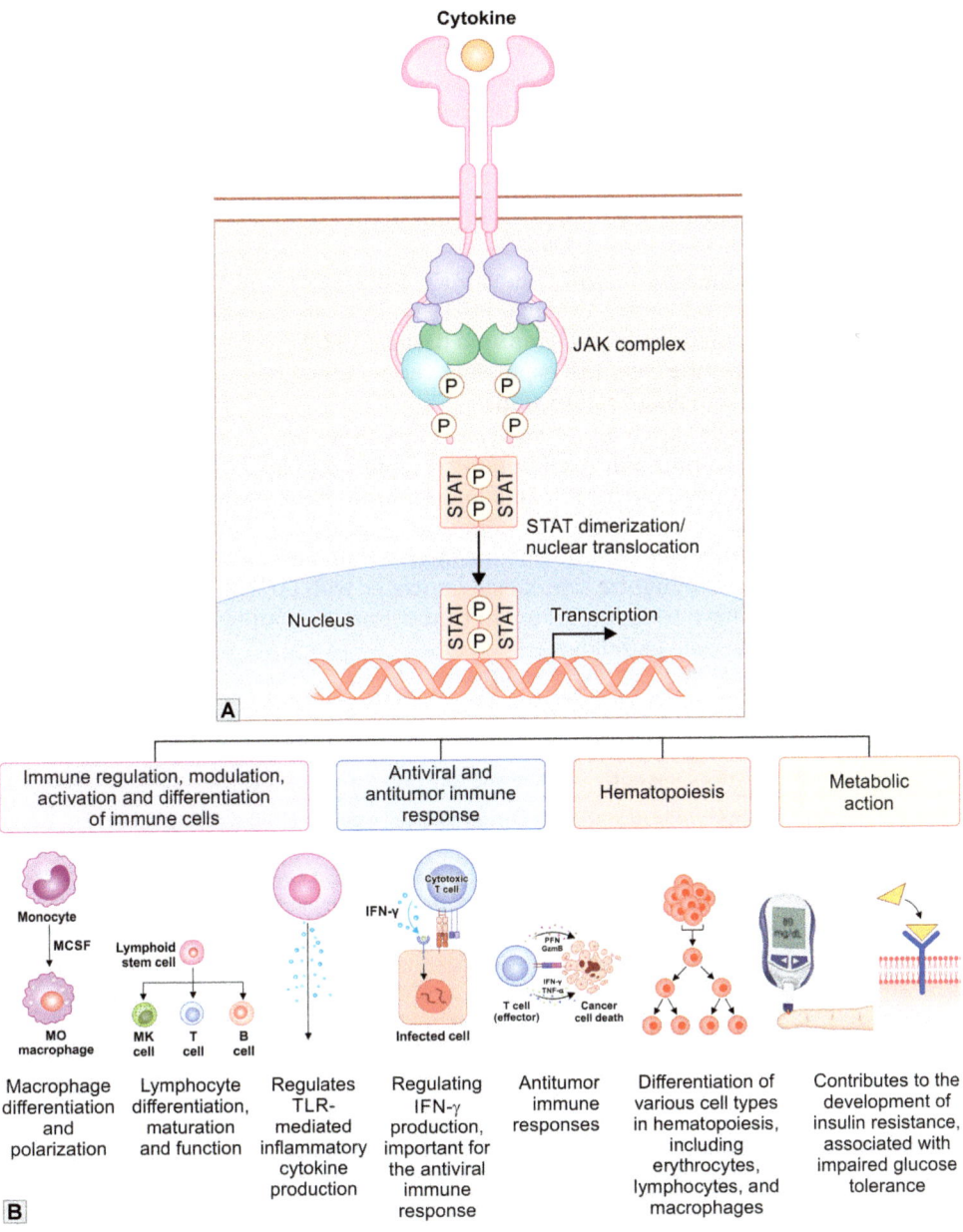

(IFN: interferon; JAKs: Janus kinases; STAT: signal transducer and activator of transcription; TLR: toll-like receptor)

FIGS. 2A AND B: On cytokine engagement, JAKs become activated and phosphorylate each other, as well as the intracellular tails of their receptors. Phosphorylation of the receptor chains generates docking sites for STATs, which can bind to the cytoplasmic domain of the receptor facilitating JAK-mediated STAT phosphorylation. Phosphorylated STATs dimerize, translocate to the nucleus, and bind to DNA, thereby regulating gene transcription. Varied functions are then mediated by the cytokines released.

kinase B (PI3K/AKT), and MAPK/extracellular signal-regulated kinase (ERK) pathways. These alternative pathways share a common feature the SH2 domain in their key regulatory proteins. This intricate coactivation pattern signifies that signaling via JAK-dependent receptors not only orchestrates the classical JAK-STAT cascade, but also instigates a more complex network of trans-signaling pathways, such as PI3K/AKT and MEK/ERK. The specificity of STAT activation is dependent on various factors and intricate regulation. These include post-translational modifications and the inhibitory function of the pseudokinase domain, as well as a large number of extrinsic regulatory elements.

Biological Functions of Janus Kinase

The varied JAK pairs mediate the function of important immune and nonimmune cells (Table 1 and Fig. 3).

The different members of the JAK family, JAK1, JAK2, JAK3, and TYK2, exhibit unique expression patterns in cell types. Although JAK1 and JAK2 are broadly expressed, **JAK3** is confined to **hematopoietic** cells and **lymphoid tissues**. TYK2, in contrast, is found in both **immune and nonimmune** cells. JAK expression varies among immune cell types, reflects their specific roles in signaling and functions.

Janus kinase 1 serves as a central mediator in multiple cytokine signaling pathways, including class II, γc receptor, and gp130 subunit receptors. By regulating interferon gamma (IFN-γ) production, it plays a critical role in antitumor immune responses. It significantly impacts immune responses, antitumor immunity, and bone homeostasis, making it a promising candidate for selective therapeutic intervention and offering an alternative to nonselective JAKinibs to minimize side effects associated with JAK2 or JAK3. Mutations and deficiencies in JAK1 have been implicated in cancer immunity and immunodeficiency in murine models and human pathology.

TABLE 1	An overview of the major immune cells and their JAK expression and function.	
Immune cell type	**JAK expression**	**Role and function**
T cells	JAK1, JAK3 (lesser extent: JAK2, TYK2)	• Crucial for T-cell receptor (TCR) signaling and development • Initiate the activation of key transcription factors (STAT) essential for the differentiation of Th1 (STAT1/4), Th2 (STAT5/6), Th17 (STAT3/5), and Treg (STAT3/5) cell subsets
B cells	JAK1, JAK3	Relay signals from the B-cell receptor (BCR) and cytokine receptors. JAK1 aids B cell development, JAK3 vital for maturation
NK cells	JAK1, JAK3 (also: JAK2, TYK2 for NK development)	Transduce signals from cytokine receptors (IL-2, IL-15). Promote NK cell development, survival, and cytotoxicity
Neutrophils	JAK expression less explored	Implicated in cytokine release via JAK-STAT signaling. Influence proinflammatory responses
Monocytes	JAK1, JAK2	Essential for cytokine and growth factor signaling. Regulate monocyte activation, differentiation, and immune responses
Inflammatory macrophages	JAK1-3, TYK2	Initiate essential transcription factors (STAT and NF-κB) to trigger the differentiation process: M1 (STAT1, NF-κB), M2a (STAT3/6), M2b (NF-κB), and M-reg (STAT3)
Dendritic cells (DC)	JAK1, JAK2, JAK3	Drive DC maturation, antigen presentation, and cytokine production

(JAK: Janus kinase; IL: interleukin; NF-κB: nuclear factor kappa B; STAT: signal transducer and activator of transcription)

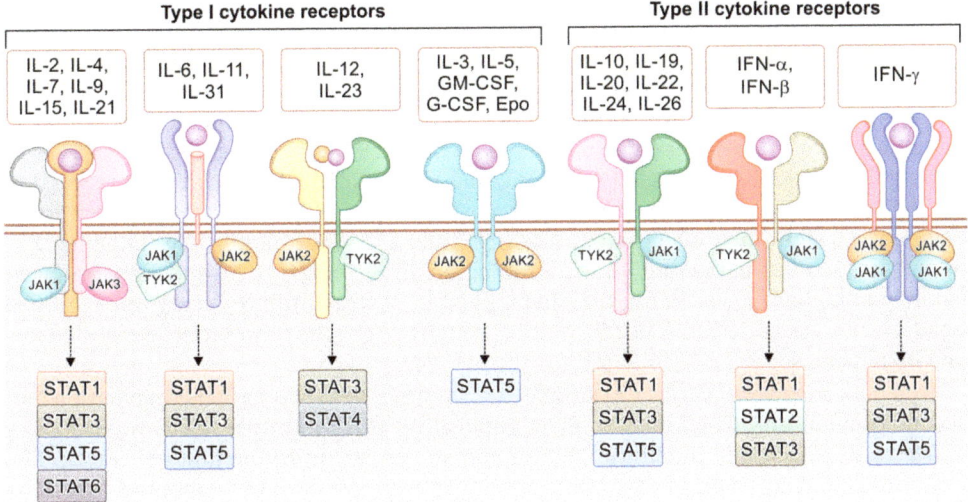

(IFN: interferon; IL: interleukin; JAKs: Janus kinases; STAT: signal transducer and activator of transcription)

FIG. 3: A depiction of the varied type I/II cytokine families and the JAK-STAT receptors that mediate their action.

Source: Bonelli M, Kerschbaumer A, Kastrati K, Ghoreschi K, Gadina M, Heinz LX, et al. Selectivity, efficacy and safety of JAKinibs: new evidence for a still evolving story. Ann Rheum Dis. 2023;0:1-22.

Janus kinase 2 plays a critical role in the signaling of type I cytokines, such as erythropoietin (EPO), interleukin 3 (IL-3), granulocyte-macrophage colony-stimulating factor (GM-CSF), IL-5, thrombopoietin (TPO), growth hormone, prolactin, and granulocyte colony-stimulating factor (G-CSF). It is essential for erythropoiesis, thrombopoiesis, and granulocyte differentiation. In particular, dysregulation of JAK2 leads to hematologic disorders, such as myeloproliferative neoplasms and leukemia.

Janus kinase 3 is crucial for the differentiation, development, and function of lymphoid cells and is a obligate partner for JAK1. It specializes in associating with the common γc receptor chain (IL-2, IL-4, IL-7, IL-9, IL-15, and IL-21), IL-3, IL-5, and GM-CSF and is indispensable for lymphoid functions and hematopoietic cell differentiation, modulating proinflammatory cytokine production in innate immune cells. Furthermore, there are metabolic implications of this cascade; JAK3 deficiency correlates with insulin resistance, while variations in TYK2 and Stat6 levels are associated with metabolic disorders, such as obesity and glucose intolerance.

TYK2 is associated with various cytokine receptors including IFNAR1, IL-12Rβ1, IL-10R2, IL-23R, and gp130 [IL-6, IL-11, and oncostatin M (OSM)]. It plays a crucial role in immune cell differentiation (Th1/Th27 response), macrophages, and NK cells activity, and influences early and osteogenic lineage differentiation in mouse embryonic stem cells.

Efficacy and Classification

The efficacy of JAKinibs can be assessed either by their inhibition of the varied Th subtypes, which express JAK receptors or more accurately by their inhibition of the cytokine cell interaction. As is obvious in the **Figure 3**, many of the type I and type II families mediate their action via JAK-STAT receptors.

Janus kinase inhibitors have been found to have a similarly broad (and maybe even broader) breadth of efficacy in various indications as the TNF-α inhibitors, even though TNF-α does not signal via the JAK-STAT pathway. In fact, these drugs with their ability to inhibit multiple cytokines are very useful when a pan cytokine effect is needed, which is true for many disorders which were believed to be a mono-cytokine disease. A classic example is atopic dermatitis (AD) and RA (see Chapter 5). In the latter they interfere with IL-6 signaling, while in psoriasis (PsO), PsA, and IBD their effect is due to the suppression of the IL-23 pathway and thus inhibits the generation of Th17 cells. A cursory look at the Figure 1 will show their effect across diseases. Their side-effect profile (e.g., anemia, HZ), though, may be due to the simultaneous inhibition of signaling by IFNs and growth factors. Notably at higher doses, 10 mg two times per day of tofacitinib or 30 mg once daily of upadacitinib, the benefit-risk profile is not acceptable, thus the dose should be started low and then increased.

Based on their selectivity for JAK molecule, they are classified into first-generation and second-generation JAK inhibitors.[3] **First-generation JAK inhibitors** have low selectivity and include tofacitinib, ruxolitinib, baricitinib, and oclacitinib. The first-generation JAK inhibitors are ATP—competitive compounds. They target the JAK homology 1 tyrosine kinase domain in its active conformation. The ATP-binding pocket is a highly conserved structure. Thus, first-generation JAK inhibitors target more than one JAK member.

Second-generation JAK inhibitors are more selective. Most next-generation JAK inhibitors are also ATP-competitive inhibitors. Nevertheless, there are certain JAK inhibitors like deucravacitinib that target the JH2 domain of JAK. JAK1 and JAK2 are crucial for signal transduction by multiple cytokines, while JAK3 and TYK2 are activated by relatively few cytokines. Due to higher specificity, the next-generation JAK inhibitors *may reduce adverse events*.

The listed drugs are given in **Table 2**.

TABLE 2	Janus kinase (JAK) inhibitors by class.	
Class	**Mechanism of action**	**Drug name**
Nonselective JAK inhibitors (first generation)	JAK 1/2 inhibitors	• Ruxolitinib • Baricitinib • Jaktinib • Momelotinib
	JAK 1/3 inhibitors	• Tofacitinib • ATI-50002
	JAK1/TYK2 inhibitors	• Brepocitinib • Peficitinib
	Pan JAK inhibitors	• Delgocitinib • Gusacitinib • Cerdulatinib • Momelotinib

Continued

Continued

Class	Mechanism of action	Drug name
Selective JAK inhibitors (second generation)	JAK1 inhibitors	• Filgotinib • Upadacitinib • Solcitinib • Abrocitinib • Itacitinib • Oclacitinib
	JAK2 inhibitors	• Fedratinib • TG101348 • Pacritinib
	JAK3 inhibitors	• Ritlecitinib • Peficitinib • Decernotinib • Brepocitinib
	TYK2 inhibitors	• Deucravacitinib • Ropsacitinib

TABLE 3 Common Janus kinase inhibitors and the cytokines that are affected by these drugs.

Receptor family		Type I cytokine receptor				Type II cytokine receptor		
		GP-130 family	IL-2R CGC family	IL-12/23 family	CβC family	IL-10 family	Type I IFNs	Type II IFNs
Cytokine ligands		IL-6, 11, 27, LIF, OSM	IL-2, 4, 7, 9, 15, 21	IL-12, 23	IL-3, IL-5, GM-CSF	IL-10, 19, 20, 22, 26	IFN-α, β	IFN-γ
JAKs		JAK1, JAK2, TYK2	JAK1, JAK3	JAK2, TYK2	JAK2	JAK1, JAK2, TYK2	JAK1, TYK2	JAK1, JAK2
Downstream STATs		STAT1, 3, 5	STAT1, 3, 5, (6)	STAT3, 4	STAT5	STAT1, 3, 5	STAT1, 2, 3	STAT1, 3, 5
Inhibitors in increasing order of selectivity ↓	Tofacitinib	+++	+++	+++	+++	+++	+++	+++
	Peficitinib	+++	+++	++	++	+++	+++	+++
	Baricitinib	+++	+++	+++	+++	+++	+++	+++
	Upadacitinib	+++	+++	++	+	+++	+++	+++
	Filgotinib	+++	+++	+	+	+++	+++	+++
	Abrocitinib	+++	+++	-	-	+++	+++	+++

(GM-CSF: granulocyte-macrophage colony-stimulating factor; IL: interleukin; IFN: interferon; JAK: Janus kinase; OSM: oncostatin M; STAT: signal transducer and activator of transcription)

Table 3 shows the spectrum of action of common JAKinibs and the targeted cytokines of the major families of type I/II cytokines, which show that even the apparently selective drugs, like upadacitinib and abrocitinib, inhibit multiple cytokine lines; hence, the selectivity may not translate to a higher safety in clinical practice.

■ OVERVIEW OF SALIENT JANUS KINASE INHIBITORS IN CLINICAL PRACTICE[4]

We will attempt to summarize the salient drugs in this class with a particular focus in dermatology. A brief history of the JAK inhibitors is depicted in the Figure 4, and this is just the beginning of the journey of this class of drugs. Notably at the moment only three drugs are as yet available in India—tofacitinib, baricitinib, and abrocitinib, but many more are expected to be approved soon.

First-generation Janus Kinase Inhibitor

Ruxolitinib

This is a JAK2 inhibitor, which was made after the discovery of GOF (gain of function) JAK2 mutations in 65–97% of patients with the common myeloproliferative diseases, primary myelofibrosis (PMF), primary polycythemia [polycythemia rubra vera (PRV)], and primary or essential thrombocythemia (ET). It was the **first** Food and Drug Administration (FDA)-approved and European Medicines Agency (EMA)-approved JAKinib for the treatment of PMF. This was then further approved for varied medical indications and has been found to reduce splenomegaly and the constitutional symptoms associated with PMF even in the absence of a JAK2 mutation.

As it inhibits both JAK1 and JAK2, there is an increased incidence of viral infections in patients on ruxolitinib. Ruxolitinib is effective in treating several inflammatory conditions and was recently FDA approved for the treatment of glucocorticoid-resistant acute and chronic graft-versus-host disease (GVHD), a major complication of allogeneic bone marrow transplantation after failure of one or two lines of systemic therapy in adult and pediatric patients 12 years and older. In dermatology, ruxolitinib is approved by the FDA for the treatment of nonsegmental vitiligo (NSV) and for AD (Fig. 4).

Tofacitinib (JAK1/3 and Partial JAK2 Inhibitor)

This was the **first studied** and **FDA-** and **EMA**-approved JAKinib for the treatment of RA, showing efficacy across many patient populations, including patients *refractory* to bDMARDs, conventional synthetic (cs) DMARDs, and also patients who were methotrexate (MTX) naïve.

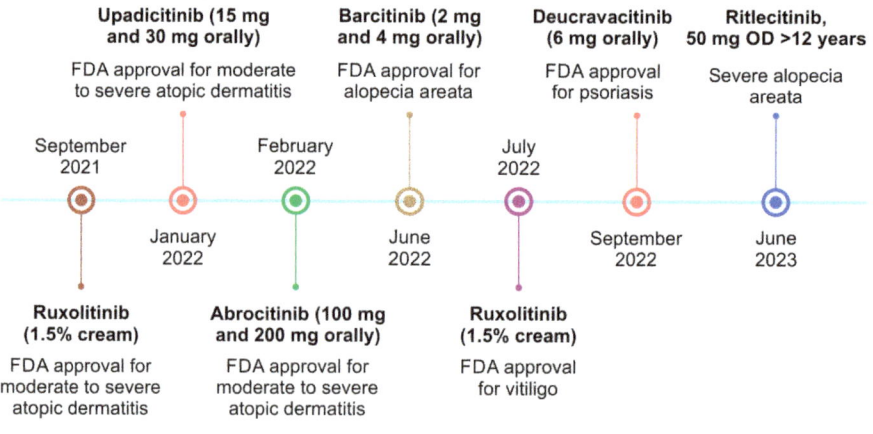

(FDA: Food and Drug Administration)

FIG. 4: Timeline of approval of JAK inhibitors in dermatology till March 2024.

While it was meant to be a selective inhibitor of JAK3, it was later noted that it also blocks JAK1, JAK2, and TYK2, although the inhibition is not uniform across these subtypes. Thus the immune cells affected include Th1, Th2 differentiation, and Th17 cells. Tofacitinib has the greatest suppressive effect on IL-6, IFN-γ, and the common γc cytokines (Fig. 3 and Table 3). In rheumatology, it has been compared with adalimumab 40 mg every other week (in combination with background MTX) showing noninferiority with the combination therapy. There is data to show its efficacy in patients with PsA with insufficient response to csDMARDs or bDMARDs and led to subsequent regulatory approval of tofacitinib for PsA.[5] It has been also shown to be effective in ankylosing spondylitis (AS) with insufficient response to nonsteroidal anti-inflammatory drugs. In patients with chronic plaque PsO, tofacitinib reduced skin disease significantly more compared with placebo treatment[6] with similar efficacy to etanercept.[7] Notably in PsO a higher dose of 10 mg BD is effective. Amongst other disorders it has been shown to be effective in systemic lupus erythematosus (SLE) and in this disorder it improves the cardiometabolic and immunological parameters associated with the premature atherosclerosis in SLE.[8] There are numerous other dermatoses where the drug is used and this will be discussed in the chapters that follow, and disorders with a prominent type I or type II cytokine profile are apt indications for tofacitinib (see Chapters 4 to 10).

The adverse events of tofacitinib are tolerable and in real world studies are restricted to opportunistic infections (OIs), gastrointestinal perforation, thromboembolism, and herpes zoster. In India a concern is tuberculosis (TB). In case of preexisting risk factors, thromboembolic events have been reported, and thus patient selection is essential (see Chapter 12). In cases of chronic viral infections such as hepatitis B virus (HBV) infection, tofacitinib therapy appears safe, but physicians should be aware of the risk of HBV reactivation. A detailed summary is given in Chapter 13.

Baricitinib (LY3009104)

This is a dual JAK1/2 inhibitor that is functionally similar to ruxolitinib and therefore suppresses IFN-γ, IL-6, IL-12/23, EPO, and GM-CSF signaling (Table 3). Baricitinib was approved for treatment of patients with RA in the 4 mg dose by the EMA and 2 mg dose by the FDA based on various studies. It has been further approved for alopecia areata (AA) and AD (Fig. 4).

The side effects seem to be similar to tofacitinib and the most common is dose-dependent increased low-density lipoprotein (42.1%), followed by an increased risk of infections, including herpes zoster and TB reactivation. A detailed summary is given in Chapter 13.

Next-generation JAKinibs and the Selectivity Paradigm

The side effects of JAKinibs are both predictable and perplexing, but to some degree can be attributed to their lack of selectivity. Tofacitinib was designed as a selective JAK3 inhibitor, yet its inhibition of JAK2 contributes to the unwanted side effects of anemia and neutropenia. Conversely, the JAK2 inhibitor, ruxolitinib, designed to inhibit bone marrow overproduction of myeloid cells, inhibits JAK1 contributing to the observed side effects.

As each JAK inhibitor impedes the combination of a JAK enzyme with ATP through the highly selective ATP-binding pocket (Fig. 2), the Michaelis equilibrium of ATP, JAK enzyme, and JAK inhibition suggests that the combination of JAK with its substrate is affected by the intracellular drug concentration and drug selectivity. The drug concentrations in turn depends on multiple factors, such as the patient's age, bodyweight, liver and renal function, and drug interactions, and it has been challenging to achieve absolute selectivity in terms of JAK inhibitors.[9]

Thus, the current experimental data does not allow us to arrive at a clear conclusion of the potential advantages of a higher selectivity of next-generation JAKinibs. One still needs to learn which beneficial effects and which adverse events are associated with specific JAKinib characteristics. Thus, additional comparative experimental data of pan and selective JAKinibs on ex vivo isolated cells from clinical trial participants are needed apart from head-to-head comparisons of JAKinibs with presumed differences in selectivity to understand the impact on safety and also efficacy. We must remember that in vitro selectivity does not translate into higher effectiveness or safety in vivo. It is important thus, to avoid being overwhelmed by industry data on selective JAK inhibitors without a head to head study.

Upadacitinib (ABT 494)

It is a putatively selective JAK1/2 inhibitor, which has shown consistent efficacy results for RA, PsA, AS, juvenile idiopathic arthritis (JIA), and IBD. It inhibits JAK1-dependent cytokines, including IL-6, OSM, IL-2, and IFN-γ (**Table 3**). In a dose of 15 mg OD, it has been approved for the treatment of RA, PsA, AS, ulcerative colitis (UC), and AD, with currently pending approval for Crohn's disease (CD). In PsA in a dose of 15 mg with MTX, it has been found to be superior to adalimumab 40 mg every other week (+MTX) in MTX nonresponding patients. Also in patients with PsA with insufficient response to non-bDMARDs, upadacitinib 15 mg and 30 mg once daily were superior to placebo treatment, with upadacitinib 15 mg once daily being noninferior to adalimumab 40 mg every other week. Also upadacitinib 30 mg once daily was found to be statistically superior to adalimumab. In AD the drug has been shown to be superior to dupilumab in a dose of 30 mg and would possibly make it more cost effective.[10] Common adverse events are infections, dyslipidemia, deranged CPK, and raised hepatic aminotransferase, followed by a reduction in neutrophil and lymphocyte counts.

Abrocitinib (PF-04965842)

This is a selective JAK1 inhibitor, which has recently been approved by the FDA for the treatment of adults living with refractory, moderate-to-severe AD. It has been shown to be comparable in efficacy to dupilumab and now an extended study up to 92 weeks has been undertaken with abrocitinib for AD. Headache, diarrhea, nausea, upper respiratory tract infection (URTI), hematologic abnormalities, and nasopharyngitis are the most common adverse events. It has been approved for use in India.

Filgotinib (GLPG0634)

This is a designed selective JAK1 inhibitor, has demonstrated efficacy for RA and UC. A recent paper described its potential use in AA.[11] It affects the Th1, Th2, and Th17 differentiation, and JAK1-dependent cytokines in a dose-dependent manner, including IL-2, IL-4, and IL-6, which plays vital pathological roles in chronic inflammation and autoimmune disorder. The common adverse events are nasopharyngitis, headache, and upper respiratory infections.

Ritlecitinib (PF-06651600)

This selective JAK3 and TEC tyrosine kinase family inhibitor has been approved in severe AA[12] and shows potential in vitiligo where it significantly downregulated proinflammatory biomarkers and increased melanocyte products in skin and blood of participants with NSV.[13] Notably tofacitinib being a JAK1/3 inhibitor would be logic be as effective in AA which is borne out by its extensive use in India.

Decernotinib (VX-509)

This selective JAK3 inhibitor was limited by multiple drug interactions, since it is metabolized by aldehyde oxidase to a metabolite that inhibits CYP3A4, which is essential for inactivation of many common drugs; hence, it is not being actively researched.

Deucravacitinib (BMS-986165)

This is the first compound that targets the pseudokinase domain of a JAK, namely TYK2, and therefore represents a highly selective, allosteric TYK2 inhibitor that can inhibit IL-12, IL-23, and IFN signaling. Deucravacitinib was superior to placebo and apremilast treatment and in a meta-analysis was also found to be superior to MTX.[14] It has also been used in LE and AA.

Brepocitinib

The drug targets TYK2 and JAK1 selectively and was efficacious in phase II studies in patients with chronic plaque PsO and AA.

An overview of the approvals of the salient JAKinib is listed in **Table 4**.

There have been, in recent years, several independently developed Chinese JAK inhibitors (e.g., including Jaktinib, golidocitinib, ivarmacitinib, and itacitinib) under different phases of clinical trials and are being considered to have great clinical potential. In October 2022, Jaktinib, a deuterated compound of momelotinib that widely inhibits JAK1, JAK2, JAK3, TYK2, and ACVR1, became the first approved domestic JAK inhibitor for the treatment of myelofibrosis.[15]

TABLE 4	Approved indications of various JAK inhibitors.
JAK inhibitor	**Approved* indications**
Tofacitinib	• Moderate to severe active rheumatoid arthritis • Psoriatic arthritis (US and EMA) • Ulcerative colitis • Juvenile idiopathic arthritis (>2 years) • Ankylosing spondylitis
Baricitinib	• Severe alopecia areata • Rheumatoid arthritis • COVID-19 infection • Atopic dermatitis (EMA and US FDA)
Ruxolitinib	*Topical*: • Atopic dermatitis (1.5% cream) • Nonsegmental vitiligo (1.5% cream) *Oral*: • Polycythemia vera • Myelofibrosis • Refractory acute graft-versus-host disease • Chronic graft-versus-host disease

Continued

Continued

JAK inhibitor	Approved* indications
Abrocitinib	Moderate to severe atopic dermatitis
Upadacitinib	• Moderate to severe rheumatoid arthritis • Psoriatic arthritis • Ankylosing spondylitis • Ulcerative colitis • Axial spondyloarthritis • Atopic dermatitis (EMA)
Delgocitinib	*Topical*: Atopic dermatitis 0.5% ointment (Japan)
Fedratinib	High-risk primary/secondary myelofibrosis
Filgotinib	Moderate to severe rheumatoid arthritis (Japan and EMA)
Pacritinib	Myelofibrosis
Peficitinib	Rheumatoid arthritis (Japan)
Deucravacitinib	Adults with moderate-to-severe plaque psoriasis (US and Japan)

*US-FDA-approved indications are mentioned, unless specified in brackets.

(EMA: European Medicines Agency; JAK: Janus kinase; US FDA: United States Food and Drug Administration)

■ TOPICAL JANUS KINASE INHIBITORS

Compared with systemically acting compounds, topically applied JAKinibs potentially have certain advantages. This includes a lower risk of potential side effects due to less systemic distribution when compared with oral administration. Thus, pan-JAKinibs could be used for conditions in which systemic long-term treatment would not be an option due to safety concerns and one example is delgocitinib. But hyperkeratotic skin lesions with thick epidermal layers and scaling make compound penetration more difficult. Topical JAKinibs have been tested in the setting of a variety of inflammatory skin conditions including **AA, AD, chronic hand eczema, cutaneous GVHD, discoid lupus erythematosus, hidradenitis suppurativa, necrobiosis lipoidica, PsO, and vitiligo,** as summarized in **Table 5**. Most of the JAKinibs tested in skin diseases are applied as creams. Exceptions include tofacitinib, which is applied in an ointment and ATI-502, which has been developed as a solution.

A JAKinib with a novel three-dimensional spiro motif is **delgocitinib**, which seems to have the best efficacy in various models. Delgocitinib has gone through phase I-III studies for patients with AD demonstrating significant improvement in the Eczema Area and Severity Index (EASI) score and has been approved in Japan for the treatment of AD.[16] It has also shown favorable results in chronic hand eczema.[17] Recently, it has been shown to be useful in vitiligo and AA.

Thus, JAKinibs have the potential to become the modern anti-inflammatory topicals and seem to be as effective as glucocorticoids and may replace them in the long-term run in terms of tolerability. But, topical JAKinibs need improvements in *structure* and *penetration* to show their efficacy in the skin. In some skin diseases, hyperproliferation and/or hyperkeratosis may limit their penetration as a deep penetration to, for example, hair follicular structures may be needed.

TABLE 5	Clinical developmental stages of topical JAKinibs for skin diseases.			
Disease	JAKinib	Target	Route	Phase of development
Alopecia areata	Ruxolitinib	JAK1/JAK2	Topical	Phase II
	Tofacitinib	JAK1/JAK3	Topical	Phase II
	Ifidancitinib	JAK1/JAK3	Topical	Phase II
Atopic dermatitis	Ruxolitinib	JAK1/JAK2	Topical	Phase III
			Topical	Phase III
			Topical	Phase I (pediatric)
			Topical	Phase I
	Delgocitinib	Pan-JAK	Topical	Phase II
			Topical	Phase I
	Tofacitinib	JAK1/JAK3	Topical	Phase II
	Brepocitinib	JAK1/TYK2	Topical	Phase II
	Ifidancitinib	JAK1/JAK3	Topical	Phase II
Chronic hand eczema	Delgocitinib	Pan-JAK	Topical	Phase III
			Topical	Phase III
			Topical	Phase II
Cutaneous GVHD	Ruxolitinib	JAK1/JAK2	Topical	Phase II
			Topical	Phase II
Discoid lupus erythematosus	Delgocitinib	Pan-JAK	Topical	Phase II
Hidradenitis suppurativa	Ruxolitinib	JAK1/JAK2	Topical	Phase II
Lichen planus	Ruxolitinib	JAK1/JAK2	Topical	Phase II
Necrobiosis lipoidica	Ruxolitinib	JAK1/JAK2	Topical	Phase II
Psoriasis	Ruxolitinib	JAK1/JAK2	Topical	Phase II
			Topical	Phase II
			Topical	Phase II
	Tofacitinib	JAK1/JAK3	Topical	Phase II
			Topical	Phase II
			Topical	Phase II
			Topical	Phase I
	PF-06700841	JAK1/TYK2	Topical	Phase II
Vitiligo	Ruxolitinib	JAK1/JAK2	Topical	Phase III
			Topical	Phase III
			Topical	Phase III
			Topical	Phase II
			Topical	Phase II

(GVHD: graft-versus-host disease; JAK: Janus kinase; JAKinibs: JAK inhibitors)

SUMMARY AND CONCLUSION

Janus kinase inhibitors have a remarkable specificity, their rapid action is consequent to cytokine inhibition, which can extend to multiple families of cytokiens (**Fig. 5**). JAKinib are markedly superior in terms of rapidity of action and spectral inhibition of cytokine families, which makes them superior to most biologicals. There is a need for H2H studies of JAKinib in varied disorders that can determine the advantage and disadvantages of selective over nonselective drugs. Also there is an issue of longevity of response, which is not seen beyond 6 weeks after stopping of therapy, though this has an advantage as the side effects are largely reversible. A knowledge of cytokine expression or JAK expression is useful, based on which JAKinib can be predictively administered in many autoimmune disorders based on the predominant cytokine expression (**Fig. 3**). Notably the data that determines the JAK inhibition is based on in vitro data and high doses can override the selectivity, and thus doses may need to be kept low and gradually escalated. There is as yet no conclusive evidence that selective JAKinibs are superior to nonselective JAKinibs, and one should look beyond industry-driven data. There is also a need to understand if drugs like MTX or biologicals can be combined with JAKinib. Possibly one can use JAKinib for initial control followed by the use of biologicals for a more targeted control.

The topical or inhalational application of JAK inhibitors is another exciting area of research in multiple ongoing animal models and larger clinical trials. The intestinally

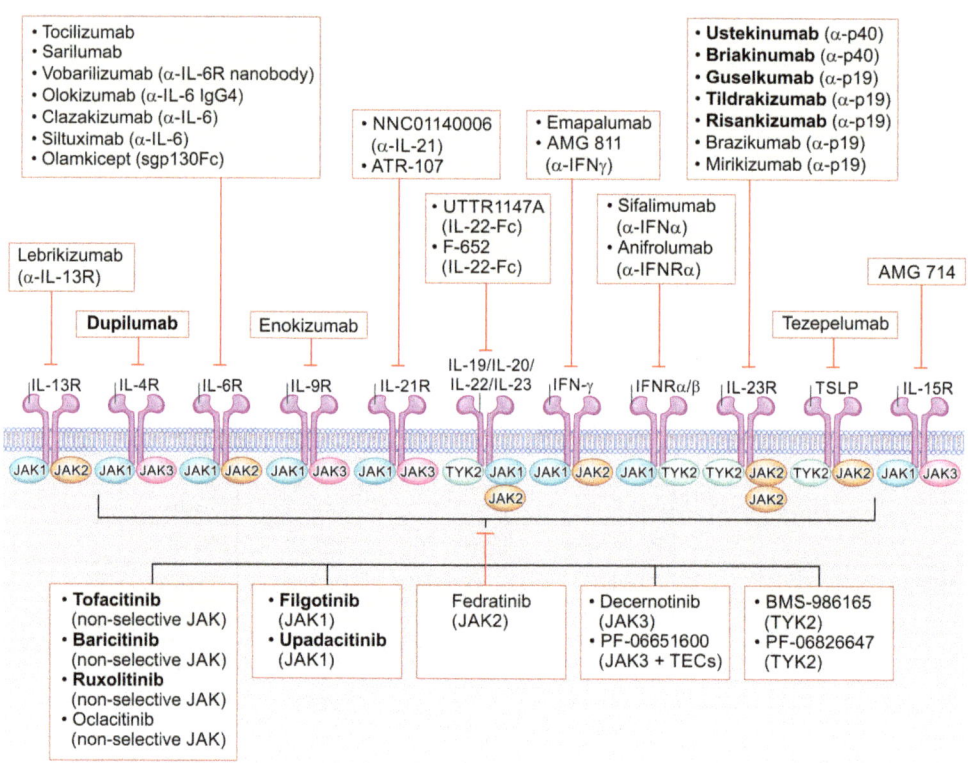

(IFN: interferon; IL: interleukin; JAKinibs: Janus kinase inhibitors)

FIG. 5: Overview of biologicals and JAKinib that inhibit cytokines. As is obvious JAKinibs have a pan cytokine suppressive potential.

restricted pan-JAK inhibitor TD-1473 is expected to soon become available to treat IBD with fewer systemic adverse side effects than other treatment options.

The ongoing development and approval of emerging JAK inhibitors in preclinical studies and clinical settings will provide optimized JAK inhibitors, which would possibly replace many of the immunosuppressive and cytotoxic agents and hopefully oral steroids which have little selective action and are a cause of multisystem side effects.

■ REFERENCES

1. Smolen JS, Aletaha D. Forget Personalised medicine and focus on abating disease activity. Ann Rheum Dis. 2013;72:3-6.
2. Genovese MC, Cohen S, Moreland L, Lium D, Robbins S, Newmark R, et al.; 20000223 Study Group. Combination therapy with etanercept and anakinra in the treatment of patients with rheumatoid arthritis who have been treated unsuccessfully with methotrexate. Arthritis Rheum. 2004;50(5):1412-9.
3. Muddebihal A, Khurana A, Sardana K. JAK inhibitors in dermatology: the road travelled and path ahead, a narrative review. Expert Rev Clin Pharmacol. 2023;16(4):279-95.
4. Hu X, Li J, Fu M, Zhao X, Wang W. The JAK/STAT signaling pathway: from bench to clinic. Signal Transduct Target Ther. 2021;6:402.
5. Mease P, Hall S, FitzGerald O, van der Heijde D, Merola JF, Avila-Zapata F, et al. Tofacitinib or Adalimumab versus placebo for Psoriatic arthritis. N Engl J Med. 2017;377(16):1537-50.
6. Zhang J, Tsai TF, Lee MG, Zheng M, Wang G, Jin H, et al. The efficacy and safety of tofacitinib in Asian patients with moderate to severe chronic plaque psoriasis: A Phase 3, randomized, double-blind, placebo-controlled study. J Dermatol Sci. 2017;88(1):36-45.
7. Bachelez H, van de Kerkhof PC, Strohal R, Kubanov A, Valenzuela F, Lee JH, et al. Tofacitinib versus etanercept or placebo in moderate-to-severe chronic plaque psoriasis: a phase 3 randomised non-inferiority trial. Lancet. 2015;386(9993):552-61.
8. Hasni SA, Gupta S, Davis M, Poncio E, Temesgen-Oyelakin Y, Carlucci PM, et al. Phase 1 double-blind randomized safety trial of the Janus kinase inhibitor tofacitinib in systemic lupus erythematosus. Nat Commun. 2021;12(1):3391.
9. Choy EH. Clinical significance of Janus Kinase inhibitor selectivity. Rheumatology. 2019;58:953-62.
10. Silverberg JI, de Bruin-Weller M, Calimlim BM, Hu X, Ofori SA, Platt AM, et al. Aggregate Response Benefit in Skin Clearance and Itch Reduction With Upadacitinib or Dupilumab in Patients With Moderate-to-Severe Atopic Dermatitis. Dermatitis. 2023. [Online ahead of print].
11. Fagan N, Doherty GA, Meah N, Sinclair R, Wall D. Cross-specialty identification of the JAK1 inhibitor trial agent filgotinib as a potential therapy for alopecia areata. Br J Dermatol. 2023;188(3):442-3.
12. Hordinsky M, Hebert AA, Gooderham M, Kwon O, Murashkin N, Fang H, et al. Efficacy and safety of ritlecitinib in adolescents with alopecia areata: Results from the ALLEGRO phase 2b/3 randomized, double-blind, placebo-controlled trial. Pediatr Dermatol. 2023;40(6):1003-9.
13. Guttman-Yassky E, Del Duca E, Da Rosa JC. Improvements in immune/melanocyte biomarkers with JAK3/TEC family kinase inhibitor ritlecitinib in vitiligo. J Allergy Clin Immunol. 2023:S0091-6749(23)01202-2.
14. Armstrong AW, Warren RB, Zhong Y, Zhuo J, Cichewicz A, Kadambi A, et al. Short-, Mid-, and Long-Term Efficacy of Deucravacitinib Versus Biologics and Nonbiologics for Plaque Psoriasis: A Network Meta-Analysis. Dermatol Ther (Heidelb). 2023;13(11):2839-57.
15. Zhang Y, Zhou H, Duan M, Gao S, He G, Jing H, et al. Safety and efficacy of jaktinib (a novel JAK inhibitor) in patients with myelofibrosis who are intolerant to ruxolitinib: A single-arm, open-label, phase 2, multicenter study. Am J Hematol. 2023;98(10):1588-97.
16. Nakagawa H, Igarashi A, Saeki H, Kabashima K, Tamaki T, Kaino H, et al. Safety, efficacy, and pharmacokinetics of delgocitinib ointment in infants with atopic dermatitis: A phase 3, open-label, and long-term study. Allergol Int. 2024;73(1):137-42.
17. Ho JSS, Molin S. A Review of Existing and New Treatments for the Management of Hand Eczema. J Cutan Med Surg. 2023;27(5):493-503.

CHAPTER 4

JAK Inhibitors in Alopecia Areata

Debatri Datta, Anupam Das

"Your hair is 90% of your selfie, do take good care of it."
—Nicole Mehta

Overview

- Introduction
- Brief Pathogenesis of Alopecia Areata
- Why Janus Kinase Inhibitors Work in Alopecia Areata?
- Overview of Treatment
- Efficacy of Janus Kinase Inhibitors in Alopecia Areata
- Synopsis of Existing Janus Kinase Inhibitor in Alopecia Areata
- Future

■ INTRODUCTION

Alopecia areata (AA) has remained a disorder, which has been largely managed by steroids, even though sadly most still persist with the use of oral steroids in its various forms, including the widely prevalent oral mini pulse (OMP). As with other autoimmune disorders, oral corticosteroid therapy represents a potential therapeutic option, but application of this modality for AA remains controversial. This is as some studies reported that oral corticosteroid administration could lead to hair regrowth, but discontinuation often results in relapse, and major adverse events can occur after the long-term use. Also it is a misused drug, and OMP in its form uses a long-acting steroid, which is inimical to the concept of intermittent steroids, and the ideal drug used should be methylprednisolone. Nevertheless the use of oral corticosteroids should be limited to a short period of time for rapidly progressive adult AA cases with hair loss, affecting more than 25% of the scalp. In the rest of cases of AA, it has no role. JAK inhibitors (JAKibs) are a more targeted approach and can replace steroids for AA.

■ BRIEF PATHOGENESIS OF ALOPECIA AREATA

Alopecia areata is a nonscarring hair loss disorder, characterized by patchy hairless areas on scalp or other parts of the body. It can be localized, or involve entire scalp [alopecia totalis (AT)] or rarely the whole body [alopecia universalis (AU)]. It is more common in young individuals <30 years of age.[1]

Hair follicles (HFs) are believed to be immune privileged sites due to their limited regenerative capabilities. In AA, there is collapse of this immune privilege, possibly due to local oxidative stress in susceptible individuals, or as a part of a dysregulated immune system.[2] Genome-wide association studies of AA have shown the upregulation of major histocompatibility complex (MHC) class I or ULBP3 (UL-16-binding protein 3) molecule, a natural killer group 2D (NKG2D) ligand in the HF, to play an important role in the pathogenesis of AA, as subsequent immune recognition initiates the attack by CD8+ NKG2D+ T cells on HFs. This results in a premature transition of anagen to catagen and telogen phases in the hair cycle, resulting in alopecia.

The follicles are invaded by CD8+ T cells and NKG2D+ cells, which identify autoantigens present in follicle roots. The salient cytokines include the interferon gamma (IFN-γ) and interleukin 15 (IL-15) (**Fig. 1**). Binding of the IFN receptors results in increased production

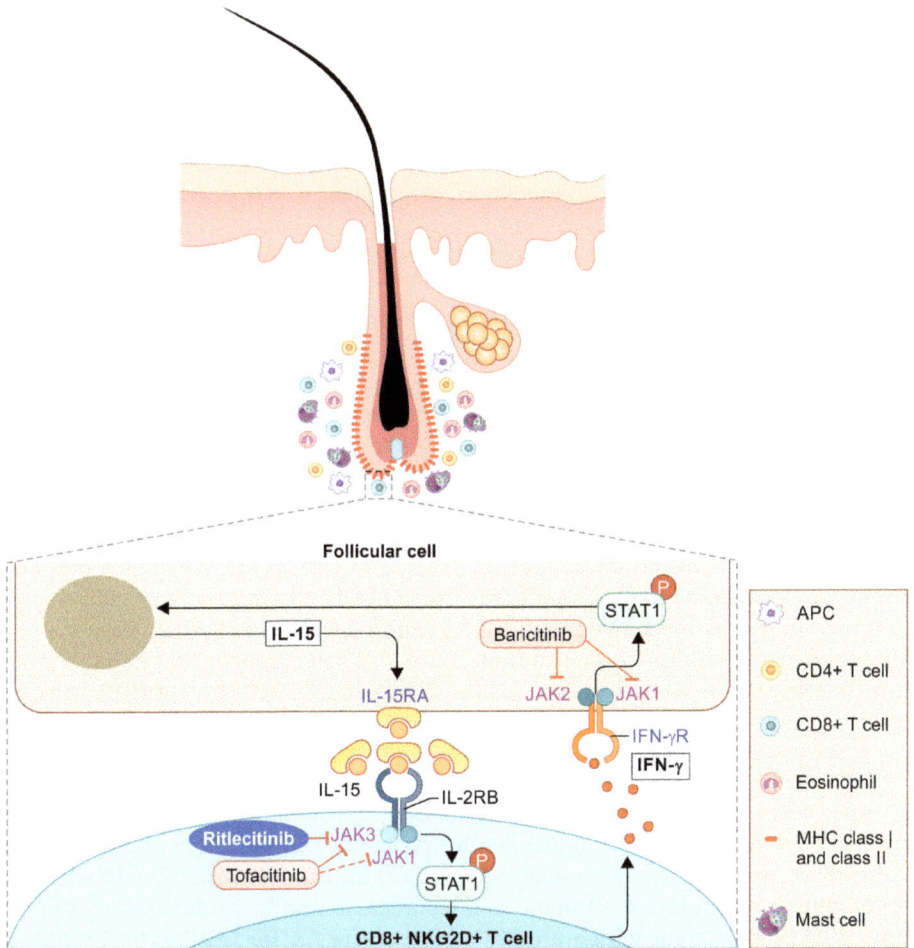

(APC: antigen-presenting cell; IFN: interferon; IL: interleukin; JAK: Janus kinase; STAT: signal transducer and activator of transcription; JAKibs: Janus kinase inhibitors; MHC: major histocompatibility complex; NKG2D: natural killer group 2D)

FIG. 1: A depiction of role of JAK-STAT pathway, immune cells, and related cytokines in the immune-pathogenesis of alopecia areata. Specific targets of various JAKibs in alopecia areata are shown in the figure. Notably, loss of immune privilege with exposure of hair follicle antigens is followed by ingress of CD8+ NKG2D+ T cell, which interacts with the follicular antigens through MHC class I. The release of IFN-γ and IL-15 leads to an autocrine loop that activates CD8+ T cells. Apart from tofacitinib, specific JAK3 inhibitors including ritlecitinib and brepocitinib have been found to be effective and hold the potential of minimizing the side effects even though the efficacy may be similar.

Source: Sardana K, et al. (2023).[5]

of inflammatory signaling molecules, including IL-15, and increased release of cytotoxic granzymes. IL-15 then activates the Janus kinase-signal transducer and activator of transcription (JAK-STAT) pathway in the CD8+ T-cells, resulting in further release of IFN-γ and thus setting up a positive feedback loop. Notably, **IFN-γ** mediates its effect via the JAK1/2 receptor and **IL-15** via JAK1/3 receptors, which forms the rationale for the use of JAKibs in AA (**Fig. 1**). It seems that IFN-γ induces the JAK/STAT signaling and thus leads to the recruitment of CD8+ T cells through CXCL9- and CXCL10-mediated mechanisms. This possibly interferes directly with the hair growth cycle via suppression of the proliferation and activation of hair stem cells and reduction of angiogenesis. This inflammation inhibits cell division in hair matrix and cause falling out of hair shafts in a telogen-type or dystrophic anagen-type effluvium.[3,4] Controlling this response can reverse the hair loss in AA as the stem cells are retained.

■ WHY JANUS KINASE INHIBITORS WORK IN ALOPECIA AREATA?

Janus kinases mediate the action of certain type I and II cytokines and are activated when cytokines and immune mediators like IFN-γ bind to these receptors. This leads to a cascade of events that leads to STAT phosphorylation, which leads to translocation to the nucleus, where it transcribes the genes of inflammatory cascade (refer to Chapter 2). JAKibs are the drugs that inhibit tyrosine kinases (TYKs) JAK1, JAK2, JAK3, and TYK2, broadly or selectively.[6]

Janus kinase inhibitors, by blocking JAK kinase pathways, can downregulate IL-2, IL-15, and IFN-γ, which are the inflammatory mediators leading to the pathological changes in AA. The **IFN-γ-JAK/STAT-IL-15** axis is the predominant player AA, which can be blocked by JAKibs, along with a possible anagen induction that leads to new hair growth.[7,8] In addition to the Th1/IFN-γ-axis, there is also a minor role of **Th2 axis**. Experimental evidence has shown that the levels of IL-4, IL-13, chemokine ligand 18 (CCL18), and thymic stromal lymphopoietin (TSLP) are increased in scalp lesions, with levels of IL-4, IL-5, IL-6, CCL17, and immunoglobulin E (IgE) and eosinophilia more prevalent in the serum/blood of patients with AA. This accounts for the association with atopy, which is a prognostic factor in AA. Recent data has found that the use of JAKibs treating patients with an atopic background may offer a positive prognosis for future development of AA. Levels of Th17-related cytokines, including IL-17 and IL-22, have also been reported to be elevated in AA lesions. Notably JAKibs inhibit all the implicated cytokines directly except Th17 cytokines.

■ OVERVIEW OF TREATMENT

A Severity of Alopecia Tool (SALT) score ≥ 20, corresponding to moderate to severe AA, is considered a general medical indication for systemic therapy. Some experts indicate a possible discordance of the recommended medical indications with available data from double-blind, randomized, controlled, multicenter, trials and with European Medicines Agency (EMA) approvals, which are limited to severe AA for JAKibs (baricitinib and ritlecitinib) and not existing for other available systemic treatment options.

The first treatment of choice in limited patchy AA is intralesional steroid injections. More widespread disease has been treated with systemic steroids, in intermittent or continuous tapering doses. Other immunomodulators like methotrexate and cyclosporine are added for steroid-sparing effects.[4] Varied other options have been tried of which topical contact allergens are the most promising. JAKibs are a new class of medicines previously used in rheumatoid arthritis, which have shown promise in the treatment of AA.[9] While various systemic agents including steroids have been used, in severe AA long-term usage is needed

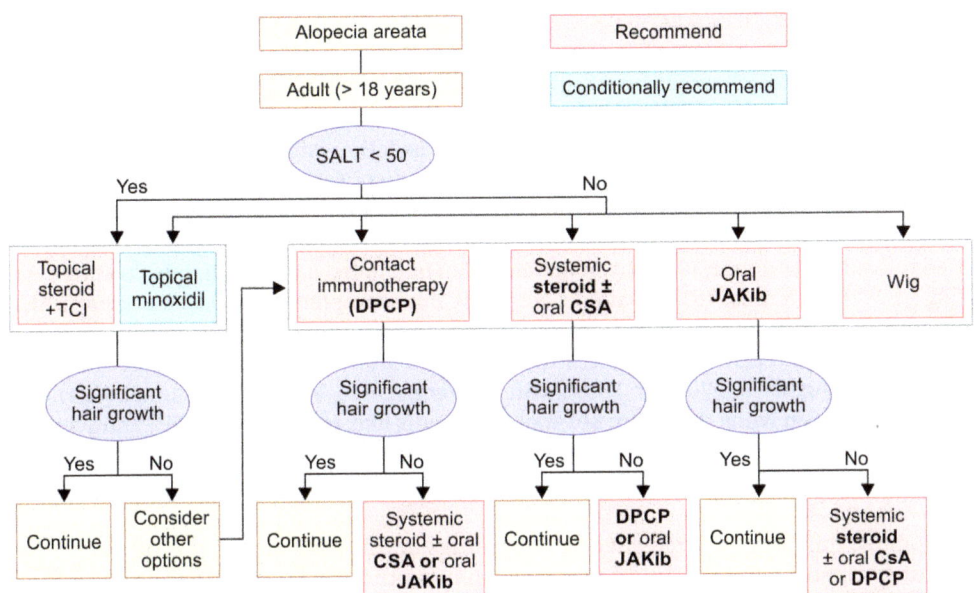

(CSA: cyclosporine A; DPCP: diphenylcyclopropenone; JAKibs: Janus kinase inhibitors; SALT: Severity of Alopecia Tool; TCI: topical calcineurin inhibitor)

FLOWCHART 1: Approach to treatment of alopecia areata and the place of JAK inhibitors (Annals of Dermatology 2023;335533:1190-204).

and in such situations it is not prudent to administer systemic glucocorticosteroids (GCS), cyclosporine, or methotrexate (**Flowchart 1**).

■ EFFICACY OF JANUS KINASE INHIBITORS IN ALOPECIA AREATA

To date, only **two oral systemic therapies** have been *approved* for the treatment of AA; these include the JAK1/2 inhibitor baricitinib, which has been approved in several countries and regions including the US and Europe, and the selective JAK3/TEC kinase inhibitor ritlecitinib, which is also approved in the US and Europe. Baricitinib has been approved for adult patients (≥18 years), while ritlecitinib can be used in both adult and adolescent patients (≥12 years). It is noteworthy that the research on these two formulations was conducted by a single doctor—Dr Brett King from Yale School of Medicine.

A systematic review in 2019 demonstrated the efficacy of JAKibs in AA, especially in refractory cases like AT and AU. Oral JAKibs, irrespective of the molecule used, were more effective than topical JAKibs.[10] Oral tofacitinib is the most studied molecule, with trials and case reports showing good efficacy in AA,[11-13] with the topical form being effective to a lesser extent.[14,15] Other JAKibs baricitinib and ruxolitinib have also showed promising results.[16-18]

■ SYNOPSIS OF EXISTING JANUS KINASE INHIBITOR IN ALOPECIA AREATA

Tofacitinib[8-15]

While there is little doubt of its efficacy, this drug should be reserved for refractory cases of AA where its use has remarkable results. A study on 90 AA, AU, or AT patients on oral tofacitinib 5–10 mg with or without prednisone showed >50% regrowth in 77% of patients (evaluated using the SALT scoring system). Of the 90 patients, 20% were complete responders (>90%

reduction in SALT), whereas 56.9% were intermediate to moderate responders (51–90% reduction in SALT for intermediate responders and a 6–50% reduction in SALT for moderate responders), and 23.1% were nonresponders (≤5% reduction in SALT).[12]

Localized disease with AA and duration of disease ≤10 years had a good prognosis. The existent data reveals that this drug can be used in isolation without oral steroids, the use of which defeats the purpose of JAKib and also predisposes to more side effects. While there are numerous studies, very few look at severe therapy-resistant cases of AA, which is more relevant than placebo-controlled industry-sponsored studies. A recent Indian study[8] used tofacitinib as a monotherapy in patients who had failed a host of agents, in severe AA (SALT ≥50) with almost 76% of patients achieving near complete response. The mean SALT score prior to starting tofacitinib was 74.23, mean dose of tofacitinib used was 13.23 mg (10–15 mg), and mean duration of treatment was 9.23 months. Latest percentage change of SALT score ranged from 70.58 to 100%, with an average of 91.47%.[8] What is notable that the drug worked even when the retinue of systemic agents like, mini pulse (OMP), intravenous pulse steroids, daily oral GCS, cyclosporine, methotrexate, and azathioprine had failed (**Figs. 2A and B**). The drug has been also found to be effective in cases of pediatric AA (**Figs. 3A and B**).

Notably, this drug is as effective as other drugs in this class and as it is off patent the parent company (Pfizer) would be more keen on approvals for the other drugs in their basket namely, ritlecitinib!

Baricitinib[18]

This is an orally administered, selective, and reversible noncovalent inhibitor of JAK1 and JAK2 that was recently approved to treat adults with severe AA. Two phase three studies, BRAVE-AA1 (NCT03570749) and BRAVE-AA2 (NCT03899259), investigated the efficacy and safety of baricitinib in adult patients with ≥50% scalp hair loss. The primary endpoint for both studies was the proportion of patients with a SALT score of ≤20 (≤20% scalp without hair) at week 36. In BRAVE-AA1, 38.8% of patients receiving baricitinib 4 mg and 22.8% of those receiving baricitinib 2 mg had a SALT score of ≤20 at week 36, compared

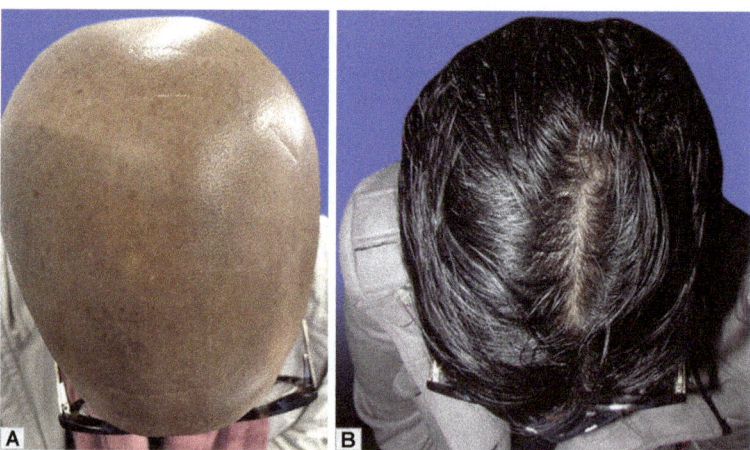

FIGS. 2A AND B: This 24-year-old unmarried female came with a wig after having tried all the oral medications including the much "acclaimed" shot gun therapy of pulse steroids both oral and IV. She was given tofacitinib 5 mg TDS and the post 6 months image reveals abundant hair. She is on the medication on an alternate-day regimen with no relapse or adverse effects.
Courtesy: Dr Kabir Sardana, New Delhi.

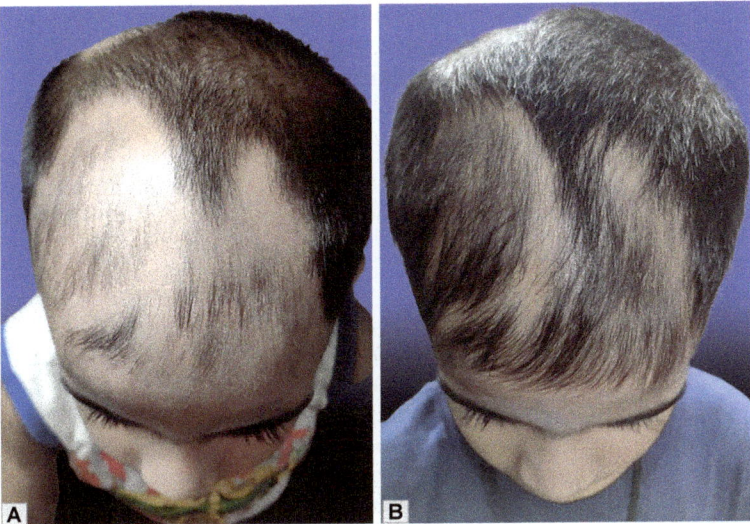

FIGS. 3A AND B: A 11-year-old boy with extensive alopecia areata progressing towards alopecia totalis. Varied options that failed included methotrexate, cyclosporine with oral steroids yielding good but short lived results. The results after 6 weeks of tofacitinib are good.
Courtesy: Dr Sujata Sengupta, Professor and Head, Dermatology, KPC Medical College and Hospital, Kolkata, West Bengal, India.

with 6.2% of patients receiving placebo; efficacy results were similar in BRAVE-AA2, with 35.9%, 19.4%, and 3.3% of patients receiving baricitinib 4 mg, baricitinib 2 mg, and placebo, respectively, with a SALT score of ≤20 at week 36. While a dose of 4 mg is used, a lower dose of 2 mg may be ideal for ≥75 years of age and for patients with a history of chronic or recurrent infections. A dose of 2 mg once daily may also be considered for patients who have achieved sustained control of disease activity with 4 mg once daily and are eligible for dose tapering and maintenance therapy. In real-world context, where patients have failed existing therapy, the results of the drug may not be marked and as JAK2 have a wide expression, drugs that inhibit this may lead to more side effects.

Ritlecitinib (Dual-target Janus Kinase Inhibitor: Targeting JAK3 and TEC)[19]

This belongs to the second-generation inhibitors that irreversibly inhibit JAK3 with >10,000-fold greater potency against JAK3 than JAK1, JAK2, and TYK2. JAK3 plays a key role in upregulation of the immunostimulatory cytokine IL-2, which regulates the opposing functions of effector cell response stimulation and maintenance of beneficial regulatory T cells (Tregs). Additionally, JAK3 does not inhibit IL-10, which potentially serves as a HF immune privilege guardian, which potentially serves as a HF immune privilege guardian. This is in addition to its effect on varied implicated cytokines of the Th1 axis, including changes to NK and T-cell activation, IL-12/23 levels, Th2, hair keratins, and hair keratin associated proteins.

This has been recently approved in June 2023 and the EMA in September 2023 for AA. A phase 3 trial lasting 48 weeks, showed ritlecitinib to be effective in treating AA and well-tolerated in patients aged 12 years and older. Doses of 30 mg and 50 mg taken once daily (with or without a saturating dose of 200 mg taken over 4 weeks) resulted in significant hair regrowth compared with the control group. The drug was generally safe. The most frequent adverse events (AEs) reported among patients receiving ritlecitinib included nasopharyngitis, upper respiratory tract infection, headache, and acne. Serious infections, herpes zoster infections, MACE, and malignancies were infrequent.

Deuruxolitinib

Deuruxolitinib (formerly CTP-543), a deuterated analog of ruxolitinib, is an orally administered selective inhibitor of JAK1 and JAK2. More data on this drug are awaited.[20]

JAKtinib

This is a deuterated analog of the JAKib momelotinib and is reported to be a stronger inhibitor of JAK2 and TYK2, compared with JAK1. Like its parent compound momelotinib, JAKib can also inhibit activin receptor-like kinase inhibitor 1 (ACVR1), a receptor of bone morphogenic proteins. Preclinical data suggest that this helps in improvement in anemia due to a change in expression of hepcidin in the liver, subsequently affecting iron metabolism. JAKib is currently under investigation as a topical cream (JAKib hydrochloride) in a dose-escalation/dose-extension (phase 1/2), randomized clinical trial in adults with AA.

Other Janus Kinase Inhibitors

The other drugs tried include brepocitinib at a dose of 30–60 mg/day (TYK2/JAK1 inhibitor), ruxolitinib (JAK 1/2 inhibitor) in a dose of 2 × 20 mg/day, upadacitinib (JAK1 inhibitor) in a dose of 30 mg/day as well as delgocitinib (JAK 1-3/TYK2) in Japan at a dose of 30 mg/day.

Janus kinase inhibitors can increase the risk of infections, especially upper respiratory infections. Increased incidence of thromboembolic events and slight increase in risk of malignancies, similar to other biologics, are seen. It is advised to do a complete blood count, biochemistry profile, fasting lipid panel, hepatitis B and C virus (HBV and HCV) serology, human immunodeficiency virus (HIV) testing, and tuberculosis screening before starting a patient on JAKibs, and monitor the parameters 3 monthly (refer to Chapter 12).[21]

■ FUTURE

Baricitinib [Food and Drug Administration (FDA) approved for use in AA], tofacitinib, and ruxolitinib are the first generation nonselective JAKibs effective in AA, with no preference in adults for either baricitinib or ritlecitinib (**Flowchart 1**). In children (aged ≥ 12 years), ritlecitinib is currently the only EMA-approved treatment. But tofacitinib has been used off-label based on its role as a JAKib and its approval for juvenile idiopathic arthritis (JIA) for age > 2 years lends way for its use in AA (**Figs. 3A and B**).[22] Although JAKibs have shown great efficacy in severe AA cases, maintenance of the results is a problem. In many cases, reducing the dose can reverse the gain from JAKibs, and stopping them altogether can even precipitate return of the original condition.[23,24] Newer selective JAKibs like ritlecitinib (JAK3 inhibitor), which have been FDA approved, may hold hope for the future.[19] Other selective JAKib molecules like brepocitinib (TYK2/JAK1 inhibitor) and deuruxolitinib (JAK1/JAK2 inhibitor) are under study.[5]

The unique aspect of this drug class is that unlike other drugs long-term usage, if needed, is safe and real world data has shown that these drugs do not have side effects even on long-term usage,[20] which is a deterrent to use steroids or cyclosporine. Guidelines have now placed JAKib as the preferred drug in their preferred treatment algorithm, which is a testimony of its safety and efficacy (**Flowchart 1**).

■ SUMMARY

Therapies that focus on targeting T-cell signaling activity are the future of therapy for AA. Till a long time, steroids were the only effective treatment option for AA. Due to possible side effects, future systemic AEs, lack of a uniform dosage regimen, and limited efficacy in severe cases like AU, steroids are usually not the preferable drug for long-term treatment. Multiple options like immunomodulators and topical contact allergens have also been tried, but none have given better results than steroids and are ineffective as monotherapies. JAKibs are a viable new option in the market for treatment of AA cases and give consistent results without the need for additional steroid therapy or having significant adverse effects and are notably the first drug class to receive approval for AA. These drugs have also shown miraculous efficacy in difficult to treat cases, giving us a ray of hope for cases with bad prognosis previously.

While outcomes of controlled trials are positive, these are against placebo which is not the ideal real-world paradigm. Thus studies that look at therapy failures are more relevant. The lack of consistent response highlights the complexity of AA immunology and reinforces the need for multiple therapeutic remedies targeting a variety of pathways involved in the pathophysiology of this disease. AA by nature is often a chronic and relapsing disease and a shifting repertoire of T-cell specificities to an ever-expanding repertoire of follicular autoantigens that emerge from repeated cycles of HF tissue disruption will further dictate the development of therapeutics targeting pathways beyond JAK/STAT signaling. This is especially true for patients with severe AA who may require multiple therapeutics with distinct mechanisms of action to achieve disease control over time with good long-term tolerance. Then there is an issue of relapse rate following withdrawal of therapy, which is still considerable, though this is true for most other drugs.

There is a need for biomarkers that can profile the severity and help to characterize treatment responders and nonresponders and assist in the development and application of immune-based therapies targeted to the specific signaling pathways involved in AA.

■ REFERENCES

1. Finner AM. Alopecia areata: Clinical presentation, diagnosis, and unusual cases. Dermatol Ther. 2011;24(3):348-54.
2. Rajabi F, Drake LA, Senna MM, Rezaei N. Alopecia areata: a review of disease pathogenesis. Br J Dermatol. 2018;179(5):1033-48.
3. Paus R, Bertolini M. The role of hair follicle immune privilege collapse in alopecia areata: status and perspectives. J Investig Dermatol Symp Proc. 2013;16(1):S25-7.
4. Trüeb RM, Dias MFRG. Alopecia Areata: a Comprehensive Review of Pathogenesis and Management. Clinic Rev Allerg Immunol. 2018;54(1):68-87.
5. Sardana K, Bathula S, Khurana A. Which is the Ideal JAK Inhibitor for Alopecia Areata – Baricitinib, Tofacitinib, Ritlecitinib or Ifidancitinib - Revisiting the Immunomechanisms of the JAK Pathway. Indian Dermatol Online J. 2023;14(4):465-74.
6. Crowley EL, Fine SC, Katipunan KK, Gooderham MJ. The Use of Janus Kinase Inhibitors in Alopecia Areata: A Review of the Literature. J Cutan Med Surg. 2019;23(3):289-97.
7. Divito SJ, Kupper TS. Inhibiting Janus kinases to treat alopecia areata. Nat Med. 2014;20(9):989-90.
8. Sharath S, Sardana K, Khurana A. A Real-World Study of Steroid-Free Monotherapy with Tofacitinib in Severe and Therapy-Recalcitrant Alopecia Areata, Alopecia Totalis, and Alopecia Universalis Cases: A Retrospective Analysis. Indian Dermatol Online J. 2024;15(1):49.
9. Darwin E, Hirt PA, Fertig R, Doliner B, Delcanto G, Jimenez JJ. Alopecia Areata: Review of Epidemiology, Clinical Features, Pathogenesis, and New Treatment Options. Int J Trichology. 2018;10(2):51-60.

10. Phan K, Sebaratnam DF. JAK inhibitors for alopecia areata: a systematic review and meta-analysis. Acad Dermatol Venereol. 2019;33(5):850-6.
11. Jabbari A, Sansaricq F, Cerise J, Chen JC, Bitterman A, Ulerio G, et al. An Open-Label Pilot Study to Evaluate the Efficacy of Tofacitinib in Moderate to Severe Patch-Type Alopecia Areata, Totalis, and Universalis. J Invest Dermatol. 2018;138(7):1539-45.
12. Liu LY, Craiglow BG, Dai F, King BA. Tofacitinib for the treatment of severe alopecia areata and variants: A study of 90 patients. J Am Acad Dermatol. 2017;76(1):22-8.
13. Kennedy Crispin M, Ko JM, Craiglow BG, Li S, Shankar G, Urban JR, et al. Safety and efficacy of the JAK inhibitor tofacitinib citrate in patients with alopecia areata. JCI Insight. 2016;1(15):e89776.
14. Cheng MW, Kehl A, Worswick S, Goh C. Successful Treatment of Severe Alopecia Areata With Oral or Topical Tofacitinib. J Drugs Dermatol. 2018;17(7):800-3.
15. Liu LY, Craiglow BG, King BA. Tofacitinib 2% ointment, a topical Janus kinase inhibitor, for the treatment of alopecia areata: A pilot study of 10 patients. J Am Acad Dermatol. 2018;78(2):403-404.e1.
16. Mackay-Wiggan J, Jabbari A, Nguyen N, Cerise JE, Clark C, Ulerio G, et al. Oral ruxolitinib induces hair regrowth in patients with moderate-to-severe alopecia areata. JCI Insight. 2016;1(15):e89790.
17. Almutairi N, Nour TM, Hussain NH. Janus Kinase Inhibitors for the Treatment of Severe Alopecia Areata: An Open-Label Comparative Study. Dermatology. 2019;235(2):130-6.
18. Jabbari A, Dai Z, Xing L, Cerise JE, Ramot Y, Berkun Y, et al. Reversal of Alopecia Areata Following Treatment With the JAK1/2 Inhibitor Baricitinib. EBioMedicine. 2015;2(4):351-5.
19. King B, Guttman-Yassky E, Peeva E, Banerjee A, Sinclair R, Pavel AB, et al. A phase 2a randomized, placebo-controlled study to evaluate the efficacy and safety of the oral Janus kinase inhibitors ritlecitinib and brepocitinib in alopecia areata: 24-week results. J Am Acad Dermatol. 2021;85(2):379-8.
20. King B. Top-line results from THRIVE-AA1: a clinical trial of CTP-543 (deuruxolitinib), an oral JAK inhibitor, in adult patients with moderate to severe alopecia areata. Milan, Italy: 31st EADV Congress; 2022. p. 3473.
21. Ismail FF, Sinclair R. JAK inhibition in the treatment of alopecia areata - a promising new dawn? Expert Rev Clin Pharmacol. 2020;13(1):43-51.
22. Sardana K, Mathachan SR, Gupta P. Pertinent role of maintenance dose of oral tofacitinib in a child with alopecia totalis with a 2.5-year follow-up on low dose. J Cosmet Dermatol. 2022;21(9):4091-4.
23. Hogan S, Wang S, Ibrahim O, Piliang M, Bergfeld W. Long-term treatment with tofacitinib in severe alopecia areata: An update. J Clin Aesthet Dermatol. 2019;12(6):12-4.
24. Haughton RD, Herbert SM, Ji-Xu A, Downing L, Raychaudhuri SP, Maverakis E. Janus kinase inhibitors for alopecia areata: A narrative review. IJDVL. 2023;89(6):799-806.

CHAPTER 5

JAK Inhibitors in Atopic Dermatitis

Kittu Malhi, Jaspriya Sandhu

"Love, the itch, and a cough cannot be hid."
—Thomas Fuller

Overview

- Introduction
- Pathogenesis of Atopic Dermatitis
- Biomarkers in Atopic Dermatitis and their Therapeutic Importance
- Overview of the Drug Pipeline in Atopic Dermatitis and Role of Janus Kinase Inhibitors
- Efficacy of Janus Kinase Inhibitors in Atopic Dermatitis
- Pharmacokinetics and Drug Interaction Profile of Systemic Janus Kinase Inhibitors
- Safety and Adverse Effects
- Expert Opinion and Conclusion

■ INTRODUCTION

Atopic dermatitis (AD) is a chronic inflammatory pruritic skin disorder marked by a remitting-relapsing course and marked patient morbidity, with the limitation of a safe and targeted treatment option.

The pathogenesis of AD revolves around a complex interplay of various genetic, environmental, and immunological factors. Barrier dysfunction and immune dysregulation skew the adaptive immune response toward the T-helper 2 (Th2) axis, giving rise to a diverse cytokine milieu.[1] The downstream signaling pathways utilized by various prominent cytokines in AD, such as interleukin 4 (IL-4), IL-5, IL-13, and IL-31, have been investigated in detail, and targeted treatment approaches are being designed.[1] Recent data has shown that there are varied endotypes of AD with a Th1/Th2/Th17 profile, which can vary over age and stages of the disease, and hence, a monocytokine inhibitor drug like dupilumab will not be consistently effective. Janus kinases (JAK) and signal transducer and activator of transcription (STAT) are a family of transmembrane receptors that participate in intercellular signaling pathways of cytokines and interferons (See Chapter 2) and by its action would block multiple cytokines pathways,[2] making it an appealing target in managing inflammatory skin disorders, given its integral role in inflammatory pathways.[2]

Various oral and topical JAK inhibitors are tested in AD for their efficacy and safety. This chapter aims to provide a brief overview of the role of the JAK-STAT pathway in AD and the utility of JAK inhibitors in the treatment of AD.

■ PATHOGENESIS OF ATOPIC DERMATITIS

Disrupted skin barrier function secondary to genetic (filaggrin mutations) and environmental factors promote allergen sensitization and polarization of the adaptive immune response. The immunopathogenesis of AD is a two-phase T-cell-mediated inflammatory process. During the acute phase, Th2-driven immune responses release cytokines (IL-4, IL-5, IL-13, and IL-31) upon exposure to allergens, thymic stromal lymphopoietin (TSLP), or IL-33, promoting local inflammation.[3] IL-4 and IL-13 are pivotal in activating Th2 cells, inducing differentiation of myeloid and atopic dendritic cells, activating B cells, promoting immunoglobulin E (IgE) class switching, and recruiting eosinophils (**Fig. 1**).[3] Clinically, these cytokines contribute to skin barrier defects, cutaneous infections, inflammation, skin thickening, and itchiness and are associated with AD disease activity.[3] IL-31 is implicated in AD-related itching and delays eosinophil apoptosis via IL-31 receptor A (IL-31RA).[4] IL-5 is pivotal in eosinophil differentiation, proliferation, and increased sensitivity to allergic reactions. In the chronic phase of AD, heightened IL-12, interferon gamma (IFN-γ), and granulocyte-macrophage colony-stimulating factor (GM-CSF) levels indicate a Th1 immune response.[5] Th17 and Th22 cytokines (IL-17, IL-19, and IL-22) contribute to persistent skin lesions, especially in pediatric, Asian, and genetically predisposed individuals.[5]

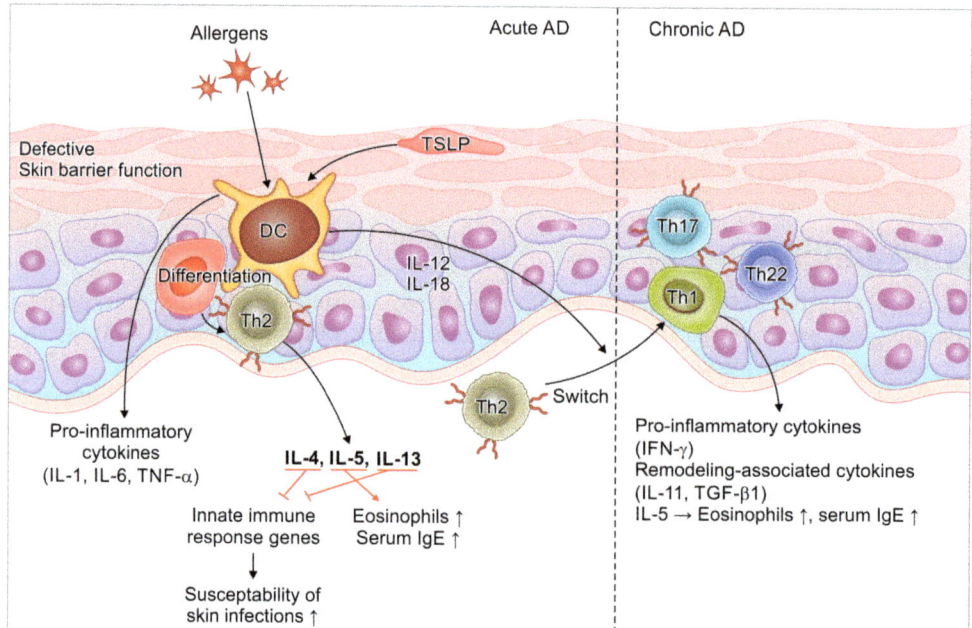

(DC: dendritic cell; INF: interferon; IL: interleukin; TGF: transforming growth factor; TNF: tumor necrosis factor; TSLP: thymic stromal lymphopoietin)

FIG. 1: Phases of pathogenesis in atopic dermatitis (AD). Genetic and environmental factors compromise the skin barrier, enabling allergens and *Staphylococcus aureus* invasion. TSLP, IL-25, and IL-33 from keratinocytes activate the Th2 response, causing barrier dysfunction in acute AD. In the chronic phase, Th17, Th22, and Th1 responses drive local inflammation and epidermal hyperplasia.

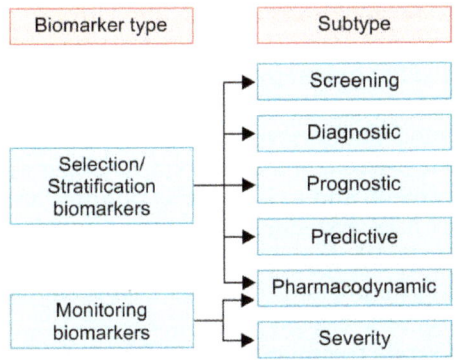

FIG. 2: An overview of the major biomarkers in atopic dermatitis (AD).

■ BIOMARKERS IN ATOPIC DERMATITIS AND THEIR THERAPEUTIC IMPORTANCE

According to the United States Food and Drug Administration (US FDA), a biomarker is "a defined characteristic that is measured as an indicator of normal biologic processes, pathogenic processes, or responses to an exposure or intervention, including therapeutic interventions." Biomarkers can be broadly separated into two categories (**Fig. 2**). The first category comprises biomarkers that are used to identify persons at risk of developing a disease (screening biomarkers), patients with active disease (diagnostic biomarkers), disease recurrence or progression in patients who have the disease (prognostic biomarkers), and the populations of patients that are most likely to benefit from a given therapy (predictive biomarkers). The second category includes biomarkers for monitoring treatment effects (disease severity biomarkers) and possible side effects (pharmacodynamics biomarkers) (**Fig. 2**).

It has become increasingly clear that not only is AD heterogeneous based on clinical characteristics but also that different underlying pathophysiologic processes can be seen in different subgroups of patients. Because of this heterogeneity, it is *unlikely* that newly developed biologic drugs targeting specific components of the immune system will be effective in all patients with AD. This is important to appreciate and has direct relevance in the treatment of AD especially in India where costs are important consideration.

■ OVERVIEW OF THE DRUG PIPELINE IN ATOPIC DERMATITIS AND ROLE OF JANUS KINASE INHIBITORS

Current guidelines for AD treatment are based on a step-up approach to therapy, which emphasizes on basic skin care (i.e., optimized bathing, moisturization, and itch-trigger avoidance) as the foundation of treatment and this has not changed even with the advent of JAKib. For **mild-to-moderate AD**, prescription of topical anti-inflammatory treatment with topical corticosteroids (TCS) and topical calcineurin inhibitors remains the mainstay of management. Crisaborole 2% ointment, a first-in-class topical phosphodiesterase-4 (PDE4) inhibitor, was approved for the treatment of mild-to-moderate AD in patients >2 years old though in India this will be hampered by its costs. There are issues with the continued use of TCS, especially with steroid phobia among patients and caregivers, which limits adherence. Topical calcineurin inhibitors are associated with a high rate of application-site symptoms (i.e., stinging and burning) and have been shown to be inferior to TCS.

For patients with **moderate-to-severe** AD, the current guidelines recommend initiation of advanced systemic therapy, which historically included phototherapy and oral immunosuppressants. Phototherapy can be poorly tolerated, infeasible, or simply too cumbersome for routine use. Systemic corticosteroids are the only FDA-approved oral immunosuppressant for moderate-to-severe AD and cannot be used continuously. Thus, there are *off-label* noncorticosteroid immunosuppressive agents, including cyclosporine, methotrexate, mycophenolate, and azathioprine, but they are hampered by variable efficacy, along with safety risks, systemic immunosuppression, and frequent laboratory monitoring, which have limited their use.

Before we address the pipeline of novel drugs it is instructive to study the **Figure 3**, which elegantly shows the place of varied agents in AD.

The era of **targeted systemic treatments** for AD was heralded with dupilumab (DUPI), a first-in-class, fully humanized, monoclonal antibody (mAb) biologic therapy that binds to IL-4 receptor α (IL-4Rα) and blocks IL-4 and IL-13 signaling, which was approved by the FDA in March 2017 for moderate-to-severe AD in adults > 18 years and has now been approved for moderate-to-severe AD in adolescents > 12 years old (March 2019) and children > 6 years old (May 2020), with additional indications for moderate-to-severe asthma and chronic rhinosinusitis with nasal polyposis. DUPI has shown excellent efficacy in multiple clinical trials and age groups, along with a favorable safety profile (consisting mainly of injection-site reactions and mild-to-moderate, reversible conjunctivitis), obviating the need for routine monitoring. But as depicted in **Figure 3**, it does not work across all endotypes of AD and is prohibitively expensive. Also lesional clearance and itch reduction are *neither uniform nor absolute* across patients. Furthermore, subcutaneous injection may not be the preferred or most appropriate method for therapy in every patient. Additional systemic treatment options are needed for moderate-to-severe AD. This brings us to the role of JAK inhibitor.

The JAK-STAT signaling pathway is a crucial intracellular signaling pathway involved in cell proliferation, differentiation, immune regulation, and hematopoiesis. Four types of JAK family proteins: JAK1, JAK2, JAK3, and tyrosine kinase 2 (TYK2) and seven types of STAT family proteins: STAT1, STAT2, STAT3, STAT4, STAT5A, STAT5B, and STAT6 are known.[2] The various relevant JAKs and STATs in relation to the pathogenesis of AD have been listed in **Table 1**. Important cytokines in AD have been highlighted in bold.

TABLE 1	Various JAKs and STATs in relation to the pathogenesis of AD.		
IL family	Cytokines involved	Associated JAKs/STATs	Specific JAK inhibitors
IL-2 family	IL-2, **IL-4, IL-13**, IL-9, IL-15	• JAK1 and JAK3 (type I IL-4R), STAT1, 3, 5, 6 • JAK1 and TYK2 (type II IL-4R)	• *JAK1 and JAK3:* Tofacitinib (oral and topical) • *JAK1 only:* Upadacitinib (oral) Abrocitinib (oral)
IL-3 family	IL-3, **IL-5**, GM-CSF	JAK2, STAT5	*No specific inhibitor; JAK1 and JAK2:* Baricitinib (oral)
IL-6 family	IL-6, IL-11, **IL-31**	JAK1, STAT1, 3, 6	• *JAK1 only:* Upadacitinib (oral) Abrocitinib (oral)
IL-12/23 family	IL-12, IL-23	JAK2, TYK2	*TYK2 only:* • Deucravacitinib (oral) • Brepocitinib (oral)

(AD: atopic dermatitis; IL-4R: interleukin 4 receptor; JAK: Janus kinase; STAT: signal transducer and activator of transcription; GM-CSF: granulocyte-macrophage colony-stimulating factor; TYK2: tyrosine kinase 2)

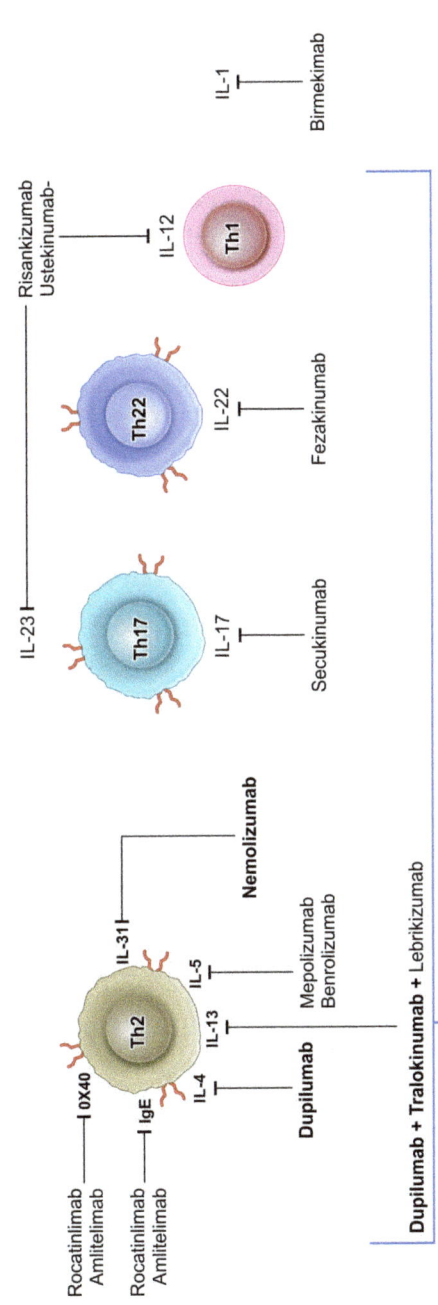

(AD: atopic dermatitis; IgE: immunoglobulin E; IL: interleukin; JAK: Janus kinase; TYK2: tyrosine kinase 2; Th2: T-helper 2)

FIG. 3: A depiction of the complex and heterogeneous pathogenetic pathways involved in AD, disease phenotypes and endotypes, and the important immunologic pathways with targeting treatments. AD endotypes can be roughly stratified into a type 2–dominant, a non–type 2–dominant, and a mixed endotype. As is obvious monocytokine drugs will not work across all subtypes which is classic of biologicals, but JAK inhibitors can inhibit multiple cytokine families.

Source: Bakker D, de Bruin-Weller M, Drylewicz J, van Wijk F, Thijs J. Biomarkers in atopic dermatitis. J Allergy Clin Immunol. 2023;151:1163-8.

Cytokine-binding induces dimerization of the receptors, causing subsequent transphosphorylation of the associated intracellular JAKs.[6] The resultant activated JAKs generate docking sites to recruit the downstream STAT family of proteins.[6] The dimerized and phosphorylated STATs are transferred to the cell nucleus and function in the transcription of various genes. Cytokines involved in the **acute phase of AD are released by Th2 cells**, IL-4 and IL-13, bind to IL-4Rs:
- Type I IL-4R (binds to IL-4) resulting in subsequent activation of JAK1 and JAK3[6,7]
- Type II IL-4R (binds to IL-4 and 13) activates JAK1 and TYK2[6,7]

Interleukin 31 is another cytokine implicated in the pathogenesis of incessant pruritus in AD. It binds to IL-31R, a heterodimer of IL-31R alpha-chain and oncostatin M-receptor chain and the ligand binding results in downstream JAK1 and JAK2 phosphorylation and subsequent intracellular signaling.[6] In case of chronic AD, the Th2 and Th22 responses are pronounced and IL-22, a key mediator of epidermal hyperplasia, binds to its receptors (IL-22R and IL-10Rb) in the skin, gut, and lungs, activating STAT3 through JAK1 and TYK2 phosphorylation.[7]

During the chronic phase of AD, **Th17 and Th22** cytokines cooperatively modulate local inflammation through upregulation of proinflammatory cytokines that stimulate epidermal hyperplasia. **Figure 3 shows** the various drugs that can be used in AD and their immunological targets. As is obvious the only drug class that can inhibit multiple cytokines and Th cell lines are JAK inhibitors.

EFFICACY OF JANUS KINASE INHIBITORS IN ATOPIC DERMATITIS

Topical Janus Kinase Inhibitors in Atopic Dermatitis

- *Tofacitinib*: Tofacitinib, a first-generation small molecule, is tailored to selectively hinder JAK1 and JAK3, with less effect on JAK2 and TYK2. In a phase 2a study for mild-to-moderate AD, 2% tofacitinib ointment applied twice daily outperformed the vehicle group, significantly changing Eczema Area and Severity Index (EASI) scores by week 4.[8] Patients using tofacitinib showed early improvements in physician global assessment, body surface area by week 1, and pruritus by day 2.[8]
- *Ruxolitinib*: It is a selective JAK1 and JAK2 inhibitor. The US FDA has approved 1.5% ruxolitinib cream for short-term and noncontinuous chronic treatment of mild-to-moderate AD in patients aged 12 years and older (September 2021).[9] In phase III, a double-blind, randomized controlled trial, topical ruxolitinib significantly improved EASI score and Investigator's Global Assessment (IGA) scores compared to the vehicle in patients with AD.[10] Treatment-related side effects are limited to nasopharyngitis and application-site pain. Topical ruxolitinib is a pregnancy category C drug.
- *Delgocitinib*: Topical delgocitinib, a pan-JAK inhibitor approved for AD treatment by Japan Tobacco, awaits US FDA approval.[11] Patients aged 2–15 and ≥ 16 years, using 0.25% and 0.5% formulations, respectively, showed higher modified EASI (mEASI) scores than the vehicle group.[12]
- *Other topical therapies in development*: Brepocitinib (BREPO), a JAK1/TYK2 selective inhibitor, is under investigation for topical and oral therapy, including AD. ATI-502 topical solution, a JAK1/3 selective inhibitor, was well tolerated in a 4-week, phase 2a OL study, with primary safety outcomes met.

Oral Janus Kinase Inhibitors in Atopic Dermatitis

- *Tofacitinib*: Oral tofacitinib appears to be a promising therapy for recalcitrant AD, with data restricted to case reports and case series. A case series involving six patients with moderate to severe AD treated with oral tofacitinib 5 mg twice daily showed a statistically significant improvement in Scoring for Atopic Dermatitis (SCORAD) scores with no reported adverse events during the 8–29 weeks. Owing to its easy availability in India, it is appealing to utilize oral tofacitinib in recalcitrant and severe AD under close monitoring.[13] Notably, the drug has the longest history of safe usage and has been approved in juvenile idiopathic arthritis (JIA) >2 years. Being a JAK1/3 >2 inhibitor, its efficacy extends to failures of selective JAK1 (see further).

- *Baricitinib*: Baricitinib is an oral JAK1 and JAK2 inhibitor approved in Japan for moderate to severe AD. A phase II double-blind randomized controlled trial (RCT) demonstrated the efficacy of baricitinib in dosages of 2 and 4 mg in the treatment of moderate-to-severe AD, with differences demonstrable in the EASI scores.[14] Two randomized phase III monotherapy trials proved significant improvement in subjective sensation of itching and rapid control of clinical symptoms in AD with baricitinib 4 and 2 mg.[15]
- *Abrocitinib*: Abrocitinib, a selective JAK1 inhibitor, is FDA-approved (2022) for refractory, moderate-to-severe AD in adults at 100 mg/day.[16] Multiple phase III RCTs confirmed the 200 and 100 mg doses of abrocitinib, alone or with topical agents, as highly effective treatments for patients aged ≥ 12 years with moderate-to-severe AD.[17]
- *Upadacitinib*: Upadacitinib, a potent oral JAK inhibitor, is FDA-approved (2022) for AD in adults and pediatric patients aged 12 years or older.[18] Recommended AD treatment: Start at 15 mg/day (12–64 years), titrate to 30 mg/day if necessary; for ≥65 years, use 15 mg/day.[18] In phase 3 RCTs (Measure Up 1 and Measure Up 2), 30 and 15 mg doses of upadacitinib exhibited significantly higher EASI and IGA responses than the placebo.[19]

Other Oral Therapies in Development

Gusacitinib (GUSA) is a selective inhibitor of JAK and SYK—a tyrosine kinase involved in signaling of proinflammatory, non-TH2 cytokines, such as IL-1b and IL-17. An early phase 1b RDBPCT suggested that GUSA is safe and well tolerated. The most common treatment-emergent adverse events (TEAEs) were headache, nausea, and diarrhea, all of which were more frequently observed in the placebo group. The drug has been granted a fast track designation by the FDA in February 2021 for the treatment of moderate-to-severe chronic hand eczema.

■ PHARMACOKINETICS AND DRUG INTERACTION PROFILE OF SYSTEMIC JANUS KINASE INHIBITORS

A thorough understanding of basic pharmacokinetic profile of widely used JAK inhibitors is a must, given their prominent utility in clinical practice. **Table 2** is a concise summary of pharmacokinetic parameters and drug interaction profile of systemic JAK inhibitors.[20]

■ SAFETY AND ADVERSE EFFECTS

Commonly reported adverse events with JAK inhibitors are typically nonserious, including upper respiratory infections, urinary tract infections, nasopharyngitis, hematological abnormalities, nausea, and headache (see Chapter 11).[20] Laboratory abnormalities linked to JAK inhibitors encompass lymphopenia, neutropenia, anemia, dyslipidemia, and elevated liver enzymes.[21] High risks of severe infections, including herpes zoster, tuberculosis, and opportunistic infections, have been associated with using JAK inhibitor in various conditions but are uncommon in dermatological practice.[21] The US FDA has issued black box warnings on approved JAK inhibitor, namely serious infections, mortality, malignancies, major adverse cardiovascular events (MACEs), and thrombosis, but it must be noted that this has been seen in a rheumatoid arthritis (RA) population who are on

TABLE 2: Pharmacokinetic profile and drug interactions of JAK inhibitors used in the treatment of AD.

Drug	Bioavailability	Plasma half life	Clearance	Drug interactions	Pregnancy category
Tofacitinib	74%	6 hours	Renal route (30%)	• *Dose reduction ↓*: Concomitant use of CYP3A4 or CYP2C19 inhibitors (e.g., ketoconazole, fluconazole) • *Dose ↑*: In case of concomitant use of CYP3A4 or CYP2C19 inducers (rifampicin)	C
Baricitinib	79%	13 hours	Renal route (69%) >> fecal route	*Atopic dermatitis*: Combination with ciclosporin is not recommended. Dose reduction in patients with concomitant use of OAT3 inhibitors (probenecid)	NA
Abrocitinib	60%	2–5 hours	Renal (85%)	Dose reduction in case of concomitant use of CYP2C19 inhibitors (e.g., fluvoxamine, fluconazole). Use not recommended in case of concomitant use of potent CYP inductors (rifampicin)	NA
Upadacitinib	75%	9–14 hours	Fecal (38%) >> Renal	• Dose reduction in case of concomitant use of CYP3A4 inhibitors (e.g., ketoconazole) • Dose increase in case of concomitant use of CYP3A4 inductors (e.g., rifampicin)	D

(AD: atopic dermatitis; JAK: Janus kinase; OAT3: organic acid transporter 3; NA: not assigned)

concomitant oral steroids and are elderly (>65 years).[21] Combining JAK inhibitors with biological disease-modifying antirheumatic drugs or potent immunosuppressants like cyclosporine, azathioprine, and methotrexate is not recommended. For monintoring see Chapter 12.

■ EXPERT OPINION AND CONCLUSION

There have been certain interesting papers that suggest that the answer to difficult AD cases may lie beyond a single drug and may require intuitive thinking and analysis of the cytokine milieu. Thus, we will examine two scenarios.

Scenario 1: A Patient Unresponsive to Conventional Steroids and Immunosuppressive Agent

The obvious choice in India would be to administer a JAK inhibitor, especially as most guidelines prefer it over cyclosporine. If one looks at the labeled indications, the ideal drug would be baricitinib, but what if this drug fails? A recent case which is one of the first cases of intraclass switching is intuitive as it looks at the role of immunology (**Figs. 4A to D) in AD**. In this case, there was initial response to baricitinib but with time the patient failed the drug. Tofacitinib was initiated and the patient responded.[23] This case highlights the

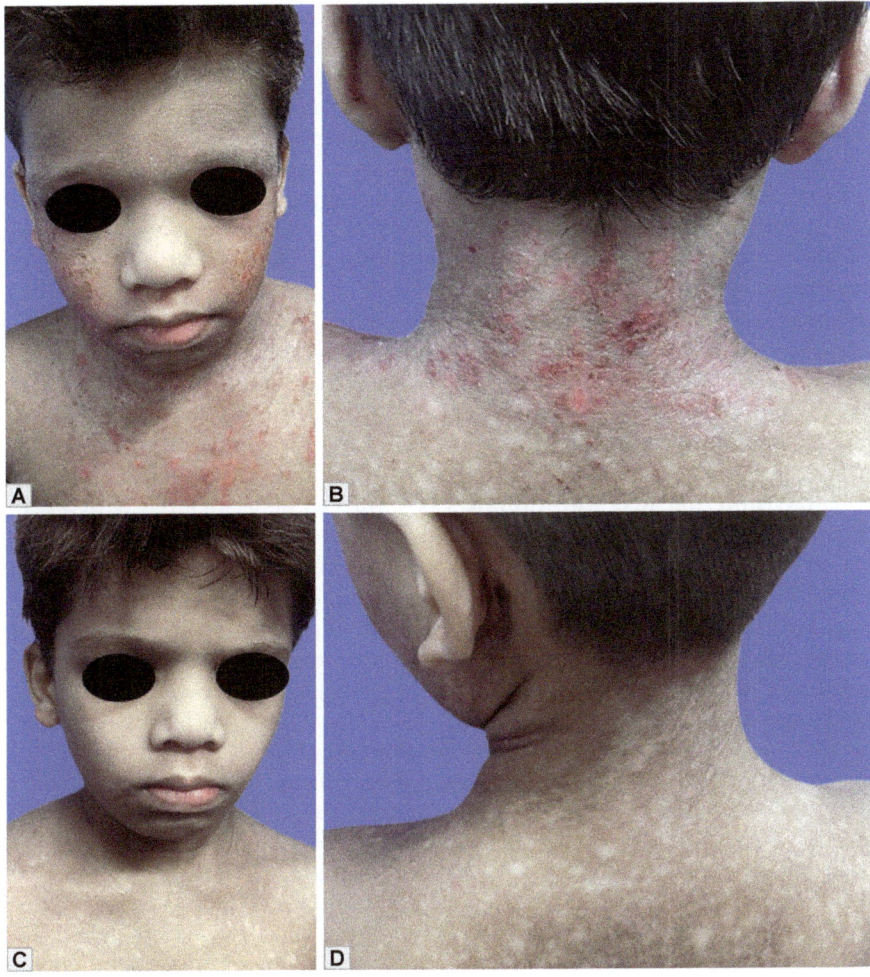

FIGS. 4A TO D: This refractory case of atopic dermatitis (AD) was initiated on baricitinib and though there was a temporary improvement the condition worsened. The drug was switched to tofacitinib with prompt control [Pediatr Dermatol. 2024 Jan-Feb;41(1):139-40.]

Courtesy: Dr Bhawuk Dhir.

aspect of tailoring the choice of JAK inhibitor for recalcitrant AD. While the predominant cellular response in AD is of the Th2 type, there is an additional role of Th17, Th1, and Th22 lymphocytes. As also shown earlier (Figs. 1 and 3), Th1/Th2/Th17 pathways play a role in the disease. IL-4 acts via JAK1/3, and IL-13 and IL-22 act via JAK1/TYK2 signaling pathways. JAKs mediate itch signaling in AD with IL-31 and TSLP, which act via JAK1/2. As multiple mediators mediate AD, the broader suppression of implicated cytokines explains the marked benefit of pan-JAK inhibitor for recalcitrant AD, which is a case for using tofacitinib, a pan-JAK inhibitor, which suppresses multiple cytokines (via JAK 1/3 signaling).

Scenario 2: Biological or Janus Kinase inhibitor?

Dupilumab, tralokinumab, and JAK inhibitors are treatment options, apart from nemolizumab. Although oral medicine is generally preferred to injection, JAK inhibitors have some safety concerns compared with dupilumab and tralokinumab. Thus, dupilumab or tralokinumab is preferred for patients who had or have risks of malignancy, cardiovascular diseases, deep vein thrombosis, pulmonary embolism, gastrointestinal perforation, or diverticulitis. Patients with renal or hepatic impairment can receive JAK inhibitors at reduced doses according to the degree of impairment, or physicians can choose the appropriate drugs considering their metabolism and excretion; however, dupilumab or tralokinumab is a better option for patients with severe comorbidities in terms of safety. Among patients treated with upadacitinib, the incidences of serious or severe adverse events and anemia were higher in elderly patients than in younger patients. Among patients treated with abrocitinib, the incidences of serious adverse events were also higher in elderly patients than in younger patients.

Therefore, in **elderly patients** and those in whom safety is prioritized, **dupilumab or tralokinumab** can be the first line as systemic therapy for AD. Age > 50 years is one of the risk factors for the development of **herpes zoster** in patients with RA treated with baricitinib. Age > 65 years and severe AD are risk factors for the development of herpes zoster in patients with AD treated with abrocitinib. Elderly patients and a history of herpes zoster are risk factors for the development of herpes zoster in patients with RA treated with upadacitinib. Because **dupilumab** was shown to be associated with a reduced risk of cutaneous infections and tralokinumab showed the same trend; dupilumab or tralokinumab should be considered instead of JAK inhibitors in patients with AD with repeated skin infections, including eczema herpeticum (**Flowchart 1**).

Janus kinase inhibitors are favored, especially for patients with a fear of needles (trypanophobia) or who prefer oral medicine to injection. Also these drugs have a rapid onset of action with a marked improvement in pruritus from 1 day after initiating the drug and rapid onset of efficacy, and they are useful in patients with severe pruritus and/or who wish for a rapid onset of efficacy. They are also preferred in patients who cannot continue systemic therapies for a long period of time owing to economic reasons; those who experience a temporary exacerbation, for instance, at a certain season; and those who need or want to receive systemic therapy over the short term for any reason. Patients with a history of conjunctivitis and/or elevated serum levels of thymus and activation regulated chemokine (over 3,000 pg/mL) and IgE (over 11,000 IU/mL) are at high risk for developing conjunctivitis during dupilumab treatment and this is another indication of JAK inhibitor. There is emerging data that shows that switching from dupilumab to a JAK inhibitor is beneficial and 30 mg of upadacitinib is superior to 300 mg of dupilumab,[24] and similar results have been noted with abrocitinib.[25] Thus, the mechanistic hypothesis of JAK inhibitors being comparable to dupilumab has now clinical evidence.

Thus in India with the high costs of therapy being a deterrent, JAK inhibitor are the ideal choice, (**Table 3**) though the use of a JAK inhibitor for > 1 year needs careful consideration owing to the lack of evidence. Here, it must be noted that prolonged use of tofacitinib up to 9.5 years[26] and baricitinib in patients with RA over a median of 4.6 years is heartening. As of now, data on the long-term use of abrocitinib for > 2 years have not been reported. Also while the safety data in RA treated with upadacitinib for a median of 4.5 years is available but in treating patients with AD with 30 mg upadacitinib on a long-term basis, we may want to consider reducing the dose to 15 mg once AD is well controlled, because the incidence of some adverse effects increased or seemed to increase in a dose-dependent manner.

Notably, there are little head-to-head studies of JAK inhibitor with the existing drugs, but clinical experience shows that the drug is effective in refractory cases of AD and thus is a cost-effective option for AD. As tofacitinib is now off patent the parent company is unlikely to perform head-to-head studies with the drug with their own selective drug (abrocitinib); hence, the real-world usage data of tofacitinib in India and its mode of action is a good reason for using it in moderate to severe AD.

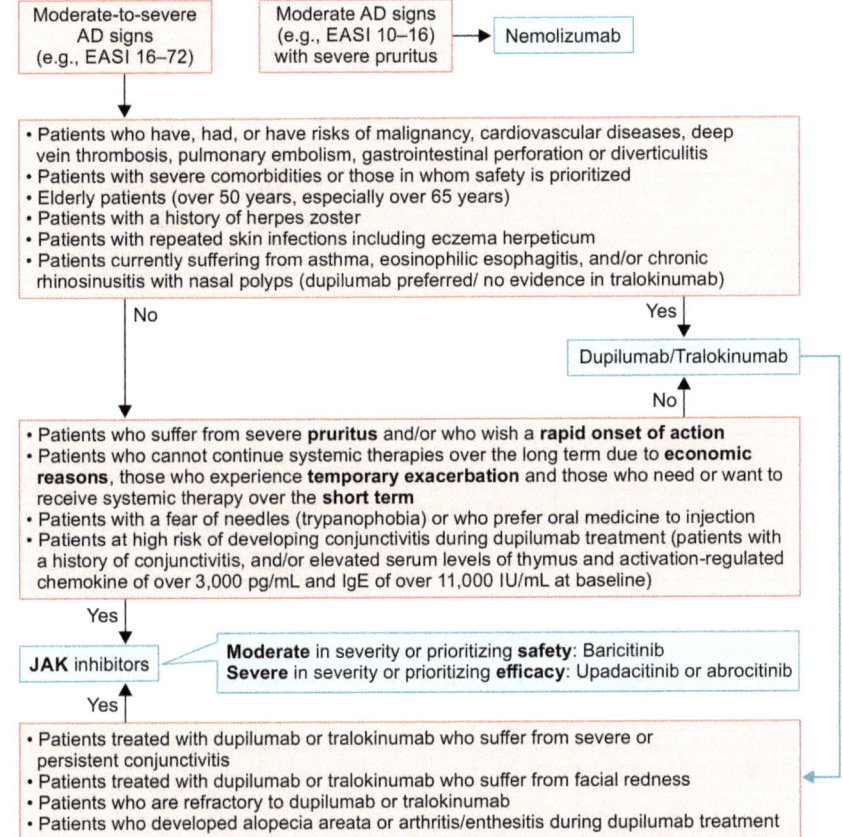

(AD: atopic dermatitis; EASI: Eczema Area and Severity Index; JAK: Janus kinase)

FLOWCHART 1: Algorithm that predetermines the choice of biologicals and JAK inhibitor in AD. Notably, cost is a major deterrent to use of biologicals.
Source: Kamata M, Tada Y. Optimal Use of Jak Inhibitors and Biologics for Atopic Dermatitis on the Basis of the Current Evidence. JID Innovations. 2023;3:100195.

TABLE 3	Summary of various JAK inhibitors used for the treatment of AD.			
Drugs	**Dosing and frequency**	**Indications and approval (if applicable)**	**Adverse effects**	**Availability**
Topical				
Tofacitinib	2% ointment twice daily	Mild-to-moderate AD	Application-site pain, pruritus, and nasopharyngitis	India, USA, and Europe
Ruxolitinib	1.5% cream twice daily	Mild-to-moderate AD in patients aged 12 years and older (**US FDA-A: 2021**)	Nasopharyngitis, application-site pain, upper respiratory tract infections, and headache	USA and Europe

Continued

Continued

Drugs	Dosing and frequency	Indications and approval (if applicable)	Adverse effects	Availability
Systemic				
Tofacitinib	5 mg twice daily	Moderate-to-severe AD, recalcitrant AD	• Nasopharyngitis, nausea, headache, cytopenia, dyslipidemia, transaminitis • Risk of serious infections (tuberculosis, herpes zoster), MACE	India, USA, Europe, and Australia
Baricitinib	2 mg once daily or 4 mg once daily	Moderate-to-severe AD	Nausea, headache, URTIs, cytopenia, dyslipidemia, increased creatine kinase levels, herpes simplex (4 mg)	India, USA, and Europe
Abrocitinib	100 mg once daily *or* 200 mg once daily	Refractory, moderate-to-severe AD in adults aged 12 years and older (**US FDA-A:2022**)	Nausea (empty stomach), upper respiratory tract infection, nasopharyngitis, and headache	USA and Europe
Upadacitinib	• Start with 15 mg/day up to 30 mg/day (age 12–64 years) • 15 mg once daily in 65 years or old	Moderate-to-severe AD in adults aged 12 years and older (**US FDA-A: 2022**)	Acne, upper respiratory tract infection, nasopharyngitis, and headache	USA and Europe

(AD: atopic dermatitis; MACE: major adverse cardiovascular events; URTI: upper respiratory tract infection; US FDA-A: United States Food and Drug Administration Approved)

■ ACKNOWLEDGMENTS

The authors thank Dr Kabir Sardana for the curated diagrams that have been modified and simplified in this chapter for easy understanding.

■ REFERENCES

1. Czarnowicki T, Krueger JG, Guttman-Yassky E. Novel concepts of prevention and treatment of atopic dermatitis through barrier and immune manipulations with implications for the atopic march. J Allergy Clin Immunol. 2017;139(6):1723-34.
2. Chapman S, Kwa M, Gold LS, Lim HW. Janus kinase inhibitors in dermatology: Part i. a comprehensive review. J Am Acad Dermatol. 2022;86(2):406-13.
3. Gittler J, Shemer A, Suárez-Fariñas M, Fuentes-Duculan J, Gulewicz KJ, Wang CQF, et al. Progressive activation of T(H)2/T(H)22 cytokines and selective epidermal proteins characterises acute and chronic atopic dermatitis. J Allergy Clin Immunol. 2012;130:1344-54.
4. Sonkoly E, Muller A, Lauerma AI, Pivarcsi A, Soto H, Kemeny L, et al. IL-31: A new link between T cells and pruritus in atopic skin inflammation. J Allergy Clin Immunol. 2006;117(2):411-7.
5. Liu T, Li S, Ying S, Tang S, Ding Y, Li Y, Qiao J, et al. The IL-23/IL-17 pathway in inflammatory skin diseases: From bench to bedside. Front Immunol. 2020;11:594735.
6. Huang IH, Chung WH, Wu PC, Chen CB. JAK-STAT signalling pathway in the pathogenesis of atopic dermatitis: An updated review. Front Immunol. 2022 8;13:1068260.
7. Furue M. Regulation of skin barrier function via competition between AHR axis versus IL-13/IL-4JAKSTAT6/STAT3 axis: Pathogenic and therapeutic implications in atopic dermatitis. J Clin Med. 2020;9(11):3741.

8. Bissonnette R, Papp KA, Poulin Y, Gooderham M, Raman M, Mallbris L, et al. Topical tofacitinib for atopic dermatitis: a phase IIa randomised trial. Br J Dermatol. 2016;175(5):902-11.
9. U.S. Food and Drug Administration. OPZELURA (ruxolitinib). U.S. Food and Drug Administration. https://www.accessdata.fda.gov/drugsatfda_docs/label/2021/202192s023lbl.pdf
10. Kim BS, Howell MD, Sun K, Papp K, Nasir A, Kuligowski ME; INCB 18424-206 Study Investigators. Treatment of atopic dermatitis with ruxolitinib cream (JAK1/JAK2 inhibitor) or triamcinolone cream. J Allergy Clin Immunol. 2020;145(2):572-82.
11. Dhillon S. Delgocitinib: First approval. Drugs. 2020;80(6):609-15.
12. Nakagawa H, Nemoto O, Igarashi A, Saeki H, Kabashima K, Oda M, et al. Delgocitinib ointment in pediatric patients with atopic dermatitis: A phase 3, randomised, double-blind, vehicle-controlled study and a subsequent open-label, long-term study. J Am Acad Dermatol. 2021;85(4):854-62.
13. Levy LL, Urban J, King BA. Treatment of recalcitrant atopic dermatitis with the oral Janus kinase inhibitor tofacitinib citrate. J Am Acad Dermatol. 2015;73(3):395-9.
14. Guttman-Yassky E, Silverberg JI, Nemoto O, Forman SB, Wilke A, Prescilla R, et al. Baricitinib in adult patients with moderate-to-severe atopic dermatitis: A phase 2 parallel, double-blinded, randomised placebo-controlled multiple-dose study. J Am Acad Dermatol. 2019;80(4):913-921.e9.
15. Simpson EL, Lacour JP, Spelman L, Galimberti R, Eichenfield LF, Bissonnette R, et al. Baricitinib in patients with moderate-to-severe atopic dermatitis and inadequate response to topical corticosteroids: results from two randomised monotherapy phase III trials. Br J Dermatol. 2020;183(2):242-55.
16. U.S. Food and Drug Administration. CIBINQOTM (abrocitinib). U.S. Food and Drug Administration. https://www.accessdata.fda.gov/drugsatfda_docs/label/2022/213871s000lbl.pdf
17. Eichenfield LF, Flohr C, Sidbury R, Siegfried E, Szalai Z, Galus R, et al. Efficacy and Safety of Abrocitinib in Combination With Topical Therapy in Adolescents With Moderate-to-Severe Atopic Dermatitis: The JADE TEEN Randomized Clinical Trial. JAMA Dermatol. 2021;157(10):1165-73.
18. U.S. Food and Drug Administration. RINVOQ (Upadacitinib). U.S. Food and Drug Administration. https://www.accessdata.fda.gov/drugsatfda_docs/label/2022/211675s003lbl.pdf
19. Guttman-Yassky E, Teixeira HD, Simpson EL, Papp KA, Pangan AL, Blauvelt A, et al. Once-daily upadacitinib versus placebo in adolescents and adults with moderate-to-severe atopic dermatitis (Measure Up 1 and Measure Up 2): results from two replicate double-blind, randomised controlled phase 3 trials. Lancet. 2021;397(10290):2151-68.
20. Eichner A, Wohlrab J. Pharmacology of inhibitors of Janus kinases - Part 1: Pharmacokinetics. J Dtsch Dermatol Ges. 2022;20(11):1485-99.
21. Le M, Berman-Rosa M, Ghazawi FM, Bourcier M, Fiorillo L, Gooderham M, et al. Systematic Review on the Efficacy and Safety of Oral Janus Kinase Inhibitors for the Treatment of Atopic Dermatitis. Front Med (Lausanne). 2021;8:682547.
22. Nash P, Kerschbaumer A, Dörner T, Dougados M, Fleischmann RM, Geissler K, et al. Points to consider for the treatment of immune-mediated inflammatory diseases with Janus kinase inhibitors: a consensus statement. Ann Rheum Dis. 2021;80(1):71-87.
23. Dhir B, Meena SK, Sardana K, Sharath S. Use of tofacitinib in baricitinib-refractory atopic dermatitis: An example of JAK inhibitor switching. Pediatr Dermatol. 2023. [Online ahead of print]
24. Blauvelt A, Teixeira HD, Simpson EL, Costanzo A, De Bruin-Weller M, Barbarot S, et al. Efficacy and Safety of Upadacitinib vs Dupilumab in Adults With Moderate-to-Severe Atopic Dermatitis: A Randomized Clinical Trial. JAMA Dermatol. 2021;157(9):1047-55. [published correction appears in JAMA Dermatol. 2022;158(2):219].
25. Reich K, Thyssen JP, Blauvelt A. Comparing how well abrocitinib and dupilumab treat atopic dermatitis signs and symptoms: a plain language summary. Immunotherapy. 2023;15(13):975-80.
26. Cohen SB, Tanaka Y, Mariette X, Curtis JR, Lee EB, Nash P, et al. Long-term safety of tofacitinib up to 9.5 years: a comprehensive integrated analysis of the rheumatoid arthritis clinical development programme. RMD Open. 2020;6(3):e001395.

CHAPTER 6

JAK Inhibitor in Psoriasis: Looking beyond Biologicals

Kabir Sardana

"Buddhism taught me that the way to change your karma is not to respond, but to feel the feeling without responding. Then it is passed on. It does no harm."
—David Guy
"Trying to Speak: A Personal History of Stage Fright"

Overview

- Brief Pathogenesis of Psoriasis
- Novel Drugs Including Jak Inhibitors
- Future Prospects

■ BRIEF PATHOGENESIS OF PSORIASIS

Psoriasis has been considered as a disease on the intersection of branching innate and acquired immunity though it is largely believed to be a type 1 T helper (Th1) disorder. The various components of the immunopathogenesis provide an integrated system of innate and acquired immunity and are depicted in **Figure 1**.

After an antigenic exposure, self-DNA is complexed with the host defense protein LL-37. LL-37 is known to enhance DNA-induced interferon alpha (IFN-α) responses in a toll-like receptor 7- (TLR7) and TLR8-dependent manner. The dendritic cells (DCs) then migrate to the lymph nodes and promote the differentiation and proliferation of Th/Tc1, Th/Tc17, and Th/Tc22 cells from naive T cells. The main cytokines that have been implicated are interleukin 12 (IL-12) and IL-23, which activate Th/Tc1 and Th/Tc17 cells, respectively. Th1 cells release IL-2, tumor necrosis factor alpha (TNF-α), and IFN-γ. The Th17 cells release IL-17A, IL-17F, and IL-22.[1] In addition to Th17 cells, IL-17 producing CD8 cells (Tc17) have been noted in the psoriatic epidermis. Th22 cells also differentiate from naive CD4 cells, and these cells are stimulated by IL-23, TNF-α, and IL-6 to release IL-22. Both IL-17A and IL-17F are considered to be relevant in psoriasis. The combined release of IL-17 release with TNF-α, IFN-γ, IL-22, IL-2, and IL-6 induces epidermal proliferation and parakeratosis and releases host defense proteins and chemokines, which induce accumulation of neutrophils, T cells, macrophages, and DCs. Persistence and disease memory of psoriasis is mediated

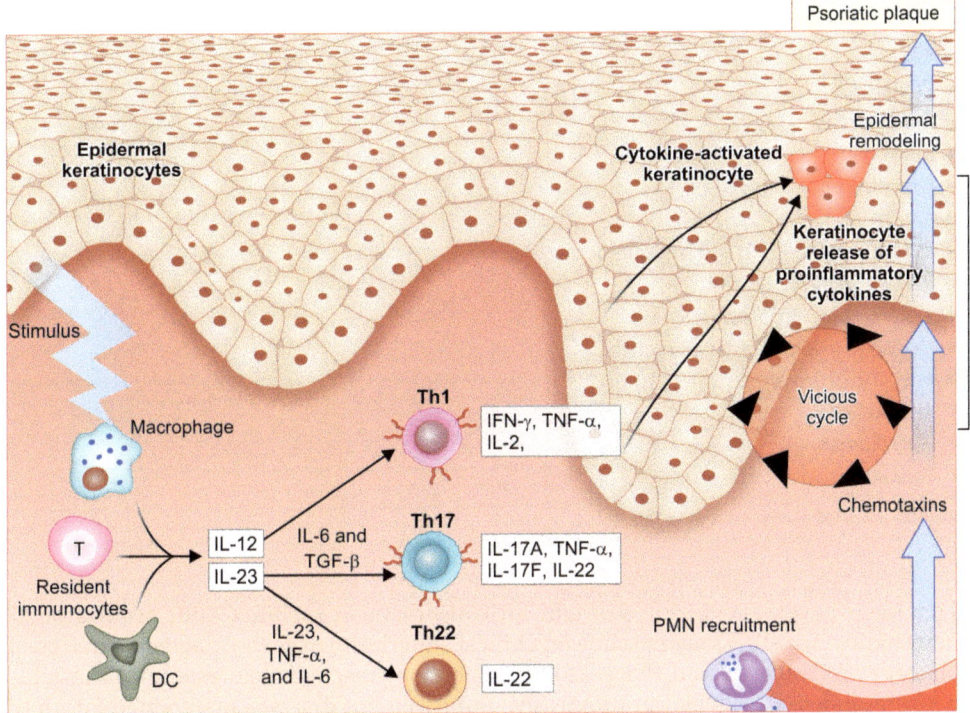

(DC: dendritic cell; IL: interleukin; PMN: polymorphonuclear neutrophil; Th17: type 17 T helper; TGF: transforming growth factor; TNF: tumor necrosis factor)

FIG. 1: An overview of the cytokine-mediated pathway in psoriasis and the dominant role of IL-12/23 which mediate the Th1 and Th17 cell, Th22 cell response, the effector cytokines of which lead to psoriasis.

by CD8+ T_{RM} cells. Recently, it has been found that epidermal cells release IL-37, which activates IL-8. IL-8 is a potent chemoattractant for neutrophils. Enhanced IL-36 signaling is a crucial pathway in pustular psoriasis. In individual patients, some segments of the pathogenesis may be more dominant than others, which may explain the heterogeneity of psoriasis when comparing individual patients.

■ NOVEL DRUGS INCLUDING JAK INHIBITORS

The biologics, which are available for the treatment of psoriasis, have been listed in **Box 1**. While long-term effective and safe control of psoriasis can be achieved with the available biologics, the results vary and they are by no means the solution as relapses do occur and biologicals can be expensive for many patients. Anti-TNF treatments achieve a 75% improvement of Psoriasis Area and Severity Index (PASI) in the majority of patients and antibodies against the IL-17 family and IL-23 achieve a 100% improvement of disease severity in about half of the patients, illustrating the relevance of the IL-23/IL-17 signaling in psoriasis. But, there are many patients that fail biologicals.

A pertinent study examined the failures on biologicals and was defined when ≥4 biologics fail to achieve a good response. The factors that predict failures include age

> **BOX 1** Biologics for the treatment of psoriasis.
>
> *Anti-TNF-α:*
> - Etanercept
> - Adalimumab
> - Infliximab
> - Certolizumab
>
> *Anti-IL-17:*
> - *IL-17A:* Secukinumab and ixekizumab
> - *IL-17A/F:* Bimekizumab
> - *IL-17 receptor:* Brodalumab
>
> *Anti-IL-12/23 (p40 chain):* Ustekinumab
>
> *Anti-IL-23 (p19 chain):*
> - Risankizumab
> - Guselkumab
> - Tildrakizumab
>
> (IL: interleukin; TNF: tumor necrosis factor)

of psoriasis onset, concurrent psoriatic arthritis, diabetes mellitus, and cardiovascular comorbidity. Anti-IL-17 agents showed clinical superiority over IL-23 agents in terms of achieving PASI 90 at 28 and 40 weeks after which they reached a plateau. In contrast, IL-23 agents showed a slower but progressive improvement that was maintained for up to 52 weeks.[2]

Due to the cost of these drugs the focus is on newer small molecules. The gene for the Janus kinase (JAK) and tyrosine kinase 2 (TYK2) proved to be susceptibility gene for psoriasis.[3] This JAK mediates the effect of IFN-α, IL-12, and IL-23 signaling. In fact IL-12/23 mediate their action via the JAK2/TYK2 pathway. This brings us to **Deucravacitinib**, a TYK2 inhibitor, which proved to be effective in psoriasis and PASI 90 was reached by 44% of the patients.[4] In comparison to other anti-JAK1/2/3 medicines, deucravacitinib is 100–2,000 times more specific against TYK2 and has limited impact on JAK1/2/3. Deucravacitinib's capacity to bind to TYK2 and form binding antagonistic confirmation between the regulatory and catalytic sections of TYK2 is what permits it to reduce TYK2 activity. The IL-23, Th17 pathway, IL-12 signaling, type 1 IFN pathway, and keratinocyte activity are all negatively affected by the downregulation of TYK2. Due to its selectivity the drug has little systemic side effects that are linked to anti-JAK1/2/3 drugs. Additionally, deucravacitinib does not affect the "IL-6 inhibition signatures" that have been seen in response to known inhibitors of the IL-6 pathway, such as JAK1 inhibitors, which can lower the level of neutrophils and raise triglyceride levels.[5]

Apart from this, other JAK inhibitors (JAKibs) have also been used in psoriasis, which include tofacitinib, baricitinib, and ruxolitinib.

FUTURE PROSPECTS

As most of the cytokines involved in psoriasis, except IL-17 and IL-36, mediate their action via JAK receptors, JAKibs as a class hold potential in psoriasis. There are various trials on various classes of drugs including tofacitinib but like apremilast we need to see their superiority over existing agents. A classic example of the futility of the so called "safe drugs" is shown by apremilast which has proved to be a safe but inexorably slow-acting drug with a recent study showing that 18.6% discontinued the drug due to lack of efficacy, 23.5% due to loss of efficacy, and 15% due to adverse reactions, and 7% due to other reasons.[6] Thus, the true test of JAKib would be in real-life scenarios where patients fail or are unable to take the existing systemic agents. In the absence of such studies, network meta-analyses (NMAs) are a surrogate marker of comparative efficacy and a recent NMA compared the drug at various points of time (weeks 10–16, 24–28, and 44–60).[7] This showed that deucravacitinib showed the highest PASI 75 response rates among nonbiologic systemic therapies across time points. Deucravacitinib PASI 75 response rate over short-term follow-up was 54.1% and was better than etanercept. At mid-term follow-up, deucravacitinib PASI 75 increased to 63.3% and at long-term follow-up, deucravacitinib PASI 75 was 65.9% and better than adalimumab and ustekinumab. Thus, this class of drug can match existing drugs and biologicals for psoriasis.

For now possibly tofacitinib may be used, which tends to work in combination with existing drugs than as a monotherapy (**Figs. 2 and 3**).

If this class of drug are able to achieve PASI 75 in a short time as compared to biologicals it would replace their use in patients who are unable to afford biologicals.

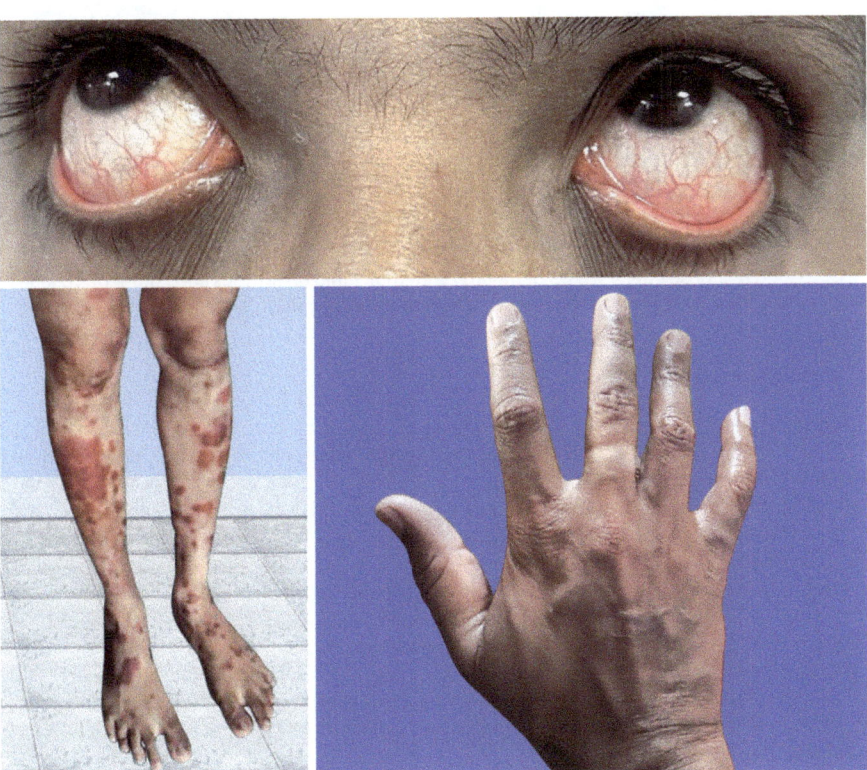

FIG. 2: Case of psoriasis vulgaris with psoriatic arthritis and uveitis with frequent relapses and poor control of arthritis even on biologics (adalimumab/secukinumab). (Dr Gautam Kumar Singh, MD Professor Dermatology).

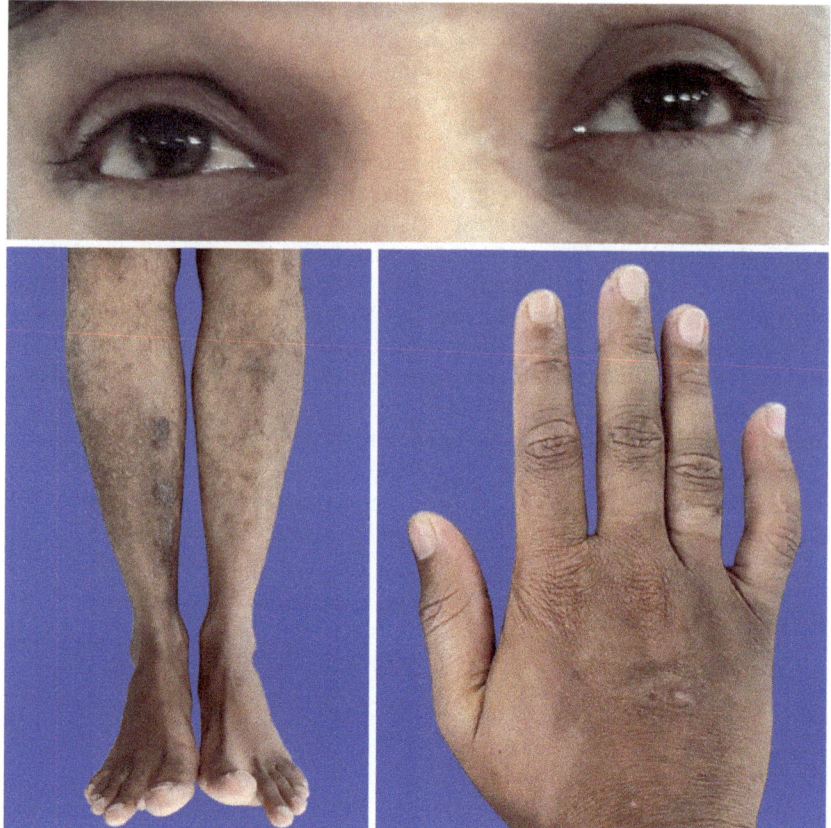

FIG. 3: Good response after 4 weeks of therapy with tofacitinib on arthritis and cutaneous psoriasis when tofacitinib was added to adalimumab. (Dr Gautam Kumar Singh, MD Professor Dermatology).

■ REFERENCES

1. Liang SC, Tan XY, Luxenberg DP, Karim R, Dunussi-Joannopoulos K, Collins M, et al. Interleukin (IL)-22 and IL-17 are coexpressed by Th17 cells and cooperatively enhance expression of antimicrobial peptides. J Exp Med. 2006;203:2271e9.
2. Viola R, Mastorino L, Megna M, Damiani G, Gisondi P. Multi-failure psoriasis patients: characterization of the patients and response to biological therapy in a multicenter Italian cohort. Int J Dermatol. 2024. [Epub ahead of print]
3. Dand N, Mahil SK, Capon F, Smith CH, Simpson MA, Barker JN. Psoriasis and genetics. Acta Derm Venereol. 2020;100:adv00030.
4. Papp K, Gordon K, Thaçi D, Morita A, Gooderham M, Foley P, et al. Phase 2 trial of selective tyrosine kinase 2 inhibition in psoriasis. N Engl J Med. 2018;379:1313e21.
5. Catlett IM, Aras U, Hansen L, Liu Y, Bei D, Girgis IG, et al. First-in-human study of deucravacitinib: a selective, potent, allosteric small-molecule inhibitor of tyrosine kinase 2. Clin Transl Sci. 2023;16:151-64.
6. Sotiriou E, Tsentemeidou A, Sideris N, Lallas A, Kougkas N, Ioannides D, et al. Apremilast Survival and Reasons for Discontinuation in Psoriasis: Five-Year Experience From a Greek Tertiary Care Centre. Dermatol Pract Concept. 2022;12(2):e2022076.
7. Armstrong AW, Warren RB, Zhong Y, Zhuo J, Cichewicz A, Kadambi A, et al. Short-, Mid-, and Long-Term Efficacy of Deucravacitinib Versus Biologics and Nonbiologics for Plaque Psoriasis: A Network Meta-Analysis. Dermatol Ther (Heidelb). 2023;13(11):2839-57.

CHAPTER 7

Janus Kinase Inhibitors in Vitiligo

Shivani Bansal, Sushama Sushama

"It's not the color of our skin that makes us different, it's the colour of our thoughts."
—Steven Aitchison

Overview

- Introduction
- Pathogenesis of Vitiligo
- How Janus Kinase Inhibitor Works?
- Efficacy of Janus Kinase Inhibitors
- Future of Janus Kinase Inhibitors

■ INTRODUCTION

Vitiligo is an acquired autoimmune disorder characterized by depigmentation due to loss of melanocytes. It has a worldwide prevalence of 0.5–1% and presents with white-colored macules.[1] There is a lot of stigma attached to this disease, which makes the patient seek treatment with the hope of achieving regimentation and stopping the progression of the disease.[2] However, there is a dearth of treatment focusing on both the abovementioned aspects of treatment. Janus kinase (JAK) inhibitors have recently gaining attention in therapeutic armamentarium in dermatology. Before assessing its efficacy in vitiligo, various facets of etiopathogenesis of the vitiligo need to be understood.

■ PATHOGENESIS OF VITILIGO

Vitiligo is a multifactorial disorder with role of both genetic and nongenetic factors. Several theories have been proposed in its pathogenesis, the most prominent of which are autoimmune, neurohumoral, autocytotoxic, and oxidant–antioxidant mechanisms, but exact cause behind melanocyte destruction is not clear.[3] Convergence theory has also been proposed, which states that oxidative stress, infection, autoimmune factors, altered environment factors, melanocyte apoptosis, and impaired migration altogether are contributing to pathogenesis.[4]

The most extensively studied is the autoimmune hypothesis in which there is abnormal cellular and humoral immunity, which leads to destruction of melanocytes. Initiation and progression of disease involves alteration in innate immunity and adaptive immunity (**Table 1**). The various cells and molecules involved have been enumerated in **Table 1**.[5]

The initiation and perpetuation of vitiligo is due to a complex interplay of epidermal cells, molecules, T-cells (including their ligands and receptors), and the interleukins (ILs)

TABLE 1	Pathogenesis of vitiligo (immune dysfunction).
Innate immunity	

Signals from epidermal cells	• Proinflammatory cytokines
	• Damage-associated molecular patterns (DAMP) including:
	  o Heat shock protein 70 (HSP70i)
	  o High mobility group protein B1 (HMGB1)
	  o Calreticulin (CRT)

Type I IFN pathway	CXCL9 and CXCL10
Inflammasome	NOD-like receptor protein 1 (NLRP1)
Adaptive immunity	
Resident memory T cells (T_{RM})	Cell surface markers: CD69, CD103, and CD49a
	T-cell homeostasis IL (IL-15 and its receptor CD-122)
	T-cell inflammation (IL-12, 18, 33, IFN-β, TNF-α)
T helper type 1 skewed profile	CD8 T cells → IFN-γ, TNF-α
	Chemokine receptor—CXCR3
	Ligands—CXCL9 and CXCL10
Cytokines	IL-17, 23, TNF-α, and IFN-γ
Signaling pathways	JAK/STAT pathway
Immune tolerance	Regulatory T cells (Tregs)
	CCL22 and IL-2

(JAK/STAT: Janus kinase-signal transducer and activator of transcription; IL: interleukin; IFN: interferon; TFN: tumor necrosis factor)

produced by them. Several pathways may act in conjunction in causation of the disease with melanocyte-specific cytotoxic CD8+ T-cells targeting melanocytes. The epidermal cells secrete heat shock protein 70 (HSP70i), which stimulates the dendritic cells to release interferon alpha (IFN-α). IFN-α induces epidermal cells to produce chemokine CXCL9 and CXCL10, which plays a role by creating a positive feedback loop for T-cell recruitment and function. Both CXCL9 and CXCL10 share a single receptor CXCR3, and it has been shown that melanocyte-specific autoreactive T-cells in patients with vitiligo express CXCR3 in blood and in lesional skin. Notably these chemokines are lined to Tc/Th1 cells line. Apart from this, there is a role of T regulatory cells (including the transcription factor FOXP3), which is responsible for stabilization of the disease, whereas resident memory T cells (TRM) are responsible for recurrence.

These cells need a favorable cytokine milieu, which includes IL-12, IL-15, IL-33, IFN-β, tumor necrosis factor alpha (TNF-α), and transforming growth factor beta (TGF-β). IL-15, signals via JAK1 and JAK3, resulting in signal transducer and activator of transcription 5 (STAT 5) activation. IL-15 has been shown to support TRM development, maintenance, and survival (**Fig. 1**).

Janus Kinase-signal Transducer and Activator of Transcription Pathway

Janus kinases, family of cytoplasmic tyrosine kinases (TYKs), aid in cytokine-mediated signal transduction through the JAK/STAT pathway (refer to Chapter 2). Various cytokines are associated with innate and adaptive responses and are implicated in vitiligo pathogenesis to mediate their action through this pathway (e.g., **IFN-α:** JAK1/TYK2; **IFN-γ:** JAK1/JAK2; **IL-2** and **IL-15:** JAK1/JAK3).[6] There is expression of IFN-stimulated genes (ISGs) by

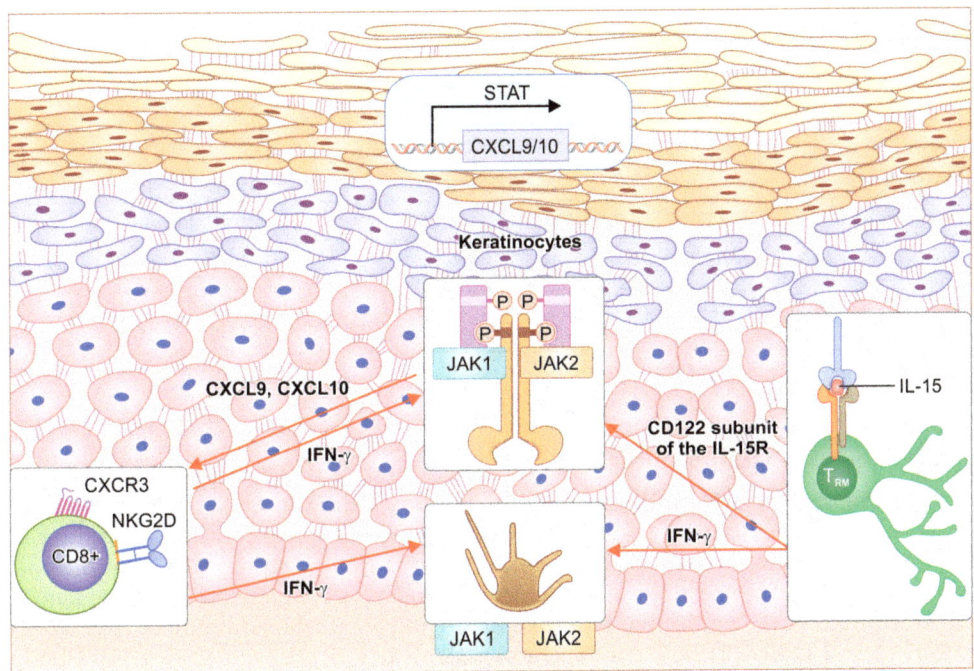

(JAK: Janus kinase; IFN: interferon; IL: interleukin; NKG2D: natural killer group 2D; STAT: signal transducer and activator of transcription; TRM: resident memory T cells)

FIG. 1: The pathogenesis of vitiligo is mediated by the NKG2D-expressing CD8+ T-cells that release varied cytokines of which IFN-γ and IL-13 mediate their action on keratinocyte via JAK1 and JAK2 receptors. There is release of chemokines by keratinocytes that via an autocrine loop activate CD8+ T-cells. The T_{RM} cells have been known to play an additional role in vitiligo via the IL-15 cytokine (modified from reference 12).

stimulation of JAK/STAT pathway.[7] **IFN-γ** is the key cytokine in vitiligo and via its receptor interferon gamma receptor 1 (IFNGR1) and IFNGR2 bind to JAK1 and JAK2, respectively. Upon binding of IFN-γ, there is dimerization of JAK1 and JAK2, which in turn leads to phosphorylation of STAT1. Phosphorylated STAT initiates gene transcription and induces the production of CXCR3 ligands CXCL9 and CXCL10 by keratinocytes. CXCL9 and CXCL10 recruit more CD8+ T cells within the skin through the CXCR3 receptor, which will produce creating positive feedback loop (**Fig. 1**).[6,8]

■ HOW JANUS KINASE INHIBITOR WORKS?

As IFN-γ signals via JAK1 or JAK2,[9] it is obvious that JAK inhibitors can block the effect of interferons. By blocking this pathway, the detachment of low E-cadherin-expressing melanocytes present in stratum basale is stopped. This step is critical before melanocyte apoptosis.[10] Also oxidative stress is known to cause relapse through IL-15 by activating the CD8+ T_{RM} cells via JAK/STAT pathway. Hence, the JAK inhibitors can help both to stop the activity of disease and also prevent relapses.[11]

■ EFFICACY OF JANUS KINASE INHIBITORS

An overview of JAK inhibitors is listed in **Table 2**.[12]

TABLE 2: Various JAK inhibitors playing a role in vitiligo treatment.

Topical JAK inhibitor		Oral JAK inhibitor	
Name of drug	JAK receptor	Name of drug	JAK receptor
Ruxolitinib	JAK1 and JAK2	Ruxolitinib	JAK1 and JAK2
Tofacitinib	JAK3 and TYK2	Tofacitinib	JAK3 and TYK2
Cerdulatinib	JAK1, JAK2, and TYK2	Baricitinib	JAK1 and JAK2
Ifidancitinib	JAK1 and JAK3	Ritlecitinib	JAK3
Brepocitinib	JAK1 and TYK2	Brepocitinib	JAK1 and TYK2
		Ropsacitinib	TYK2 and JAK2

(JAK: Janus kinase; TYK: tyrosine kinase)

Topical Janus Kinase inhibitors

Among the topical JAK inhibitors, ruxolitinib has been the most commonly used formulation followed by tofacitinib and delgocitinib.[13] Topical formulation achieves high concentration of ruxolitinib in both epidermis and dermis with little plasma concentration, and hence, there are minimal side effects as compared to oral formulation of JAK inhibitors.[14] Two double blind, vehicle-controlled trials on topical ruxolitinib (TRuE-V1 and TRuE-V2) were conducted in patients of age ≥12 years having ≤10% body surface area (BSA) of nonsegmental vitiligo of involvement, and this lead to the approval of ruxolitinib cream 1.5% for vitiligo.[15] Common adverse reactions reported in trials were application-site acne, redness, and itching. Rare adverse events were inflammation of the throat and nasal passages, headaches, urinary tract infections, and fever.[16] Other strengths of ruxolitinib such as 0.5% and 0.15% have also been found to be effective in repigmentation.[17]

Topical tofacitinib 2% has also been found to be effective for vitiligo. Although it is believed that concomitant exposure with narrow-band ultraviolet B (NB-UVB) or sun aids in the pigmentation, however authors have found results even without the exposure.[18,19] However, facial lesions and darker skin phototypes respond better than the counterpart.[19] Significant pigmentation is usually achieved by 4–5 months of application. Erythema and transient acne may be noted as a side effect of application. Delgocitinib and cerdulatinib (0.37%) gel has been used with promising results.[20,21] Various studies published on the role of topical JAK inhibitors in vitiligo are described in **Table 3**.

Oral Janus Kinase Inhibitors

Oral Tofacitinib

The use of oral tofacitinib in vitiligo was a serendipitous discovery in a female who had alopecia areata as well. She was prescribed tofacitinib 5 mg orally on alternate days initially but later was increased to 5 mg twice daily at 4 weeks. After 5 months of tofacitinib, there was decrease in depigmentation from 10 to 5% with no side effects.[22] This heralded the use of tofacitinib for localized, generalized, stable, unstable as well as refractory vitiligo with good response. However, it was noted in a study that although the CD8+ T cells decreased in lesional skin after treatment with tofacitinib, but the melanocyte specific T cells before and after treatment remained the same. This means that repigmentation needs both JAK inhibitors (for suppression of local inflammation) and light exposure (for stimulation of melanocytes) (**Figs. 2A and B**).[23] Thus tofacitinib in the dose of 5 mg twice daily along

TABLE 3 Topical JAK inhibitors in vitiligo.

Author	Type	Number of patients	Treatment	Duration (weeks)	Areas affected	Outcome	Side effects
Rosamarin et al. (2020)[15]	Double blind vehicle control trial	674 (>12 years age)	Ruxolitinib cream 1.5% BD	52	<10% BSA Nonsegmental vitiligo	TRuE-V1 VASI75 week 24—29.8% and TRuE-V2, were 30.9%	Acne, nasopharyngitis, and application-site pruritus
Rosamarin et al. (2020)[17]	Ruxolitinib cream 1.5% BD, 1.5% QID, 0.5% QID, 0.15% QID	157	Double-blinded trial	52	0.5% or more of their facial BSA and 3% or more of their nonfacial BSA	VASI 50 (week 24) 1.5% BD—45%, 1.5% OD—50%, 0.5% OD—26%, 0.15% OD—32%	Acne, upper respiratory tract infection, application-site pruritus, and headache
Mobasher et al. (2020)[19]	Tofacitinib cream 2% BD	16	Nonrandomized cohort study	N/A	Not mentioned	>90% repigmentation—4, 25–75% repigmentation 5–15% repigmentation No change—2	Acne-like papules, skin contour change

(BSA: body surface area; JAK: Janus kinase)

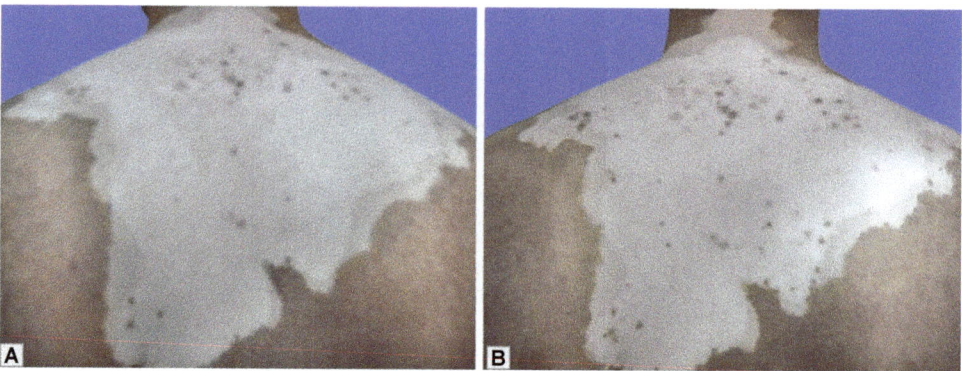

FIGS. 2A AND B: This shows a patient pre (left side) and post (right side) after 3 months of treatment with tofacitinib with minimal repigmentation but the activity of disease was halted. This shows that concomitant phototherapy is essential for visible response.

with NB-UVB phototherapy helps to induce repigmentation as early as 4 weeks with up to 75% repigmentation by 16 weeks.[24] Even low-dose tofacitinib (5 mg once daily) with NB-UVB has shown repigmentation, albeit in treatment-resistant cases where higher dose or longer duration of tofacitinib may be required.[25] Nonetheless, cases have been reported where pigmentation was seen even without light exposure.[26] Systemic side effects noted with oral tofacitinib are increased risk of infection, malignancy, hematological cytopenia, and dyslipidemia.[25] In view of these side effects, most authors have restricted the use of oral tofacitinib to 10 months even though Aickara et al.[27] have used it for a total duration of 5 years with no significant side effects. Studies which have evaluated the efficacy of tofacitinib has been mentioned in **Table 4**.

Other Oral Janus Kinase Inhibitors

Ruxolitinib in a dose of 20 mg twice daily was used in a single patient with coexistent alopecia areata and vitiligo. Although hair regrowth was retained 12 weeks after discontinuation of ruxolitinib, but pigmentation achieved was lost.[28] Similarly, baricitinib prescribed in a dose of 4 mg once daily has shown complete repigmentation in a single patient with no side effects.[29] Modest response can be seen with oral ritlecitinib in a loading dose (100/200 mg) along with daily dosing (30/50 mg) in active nonsegmental vitiligo.[30]

Trials for ifidancitinib and brepocitinib are still going on and no data is yet available. **Table 4** summarizes the various studies published on tofacitinib.

■ FUTURE OF JANUS KINASE INHIBITORS

The efficacy of JAK inhibitors has been proven through a number of case reports, case series but a limited number of case–control studies. However, many of the studies previously done have either small number of study subjects, patients of only specific ethnicity or brief follow-up. Thus, there is a need for large randomized trials with data in Indian patients where the disease is associated with high stigma. There is also higher prevalence of tuberculosis and low spending capacity, especially for non-life-threatening diseases, making it difficult to prescribe JAK inhibitors, which may appear as a cost burden to the patients. As it has been suggested[13] that these do not promote repigmentation, thus double-blinded studies with and without concurrent phototherapy should be carried out to establish its role in vitiligo.

TABLE 4 Various studies published on oral tofacitinib.

Author	Type	Number of patients / Mean age	Treatment	Duration (weeks)	Area affected	Outcome	Side effects
Liu (2017)[23]	Retrospective	10 / 54	Tofacitinib 5–10 mg daily	40	Generalized	5 of 10 patients achieved some repigmentation (three patients with sun exposed area, two patients with UVB phototherapy)	Weight gain (1), arthralgia (1), mild increase in lipids (4)
Gianfaldoni (2018)[31]	Retrospective	9 / NA	Tofacitinib 5 mg BD + UVB phototherapy	NA	Localized vitiligo	All nine patients achieved nearly complete repigmentation	Nil
Song et al. (2022)[24]	Original article	Cases 15 Control 19	• Tofacitinib 5 mg BD and phototherapy • NB-UVB phototherapy	16 weeks	Generalized	From eighth week, the repigmentation level was significantly higher in the combination group than in the controls	Seen in only one patient

(NB-UVB: narrow-band ultraviolet B)

REFERENCES

1. Elbuluk N, Ezzedine K. Quality of Life, Burden of Disease, Co-morbidities, and Systemic Effects in Vitiligo Patients. Dermatol Clin. 2017;35(2):117-28.
2. Hamidizadeh N, Ranjbar S, Ghanizadeh A, Parvizi MM, Jafari P, Handjani F. Evaluating prevalence of depression, anxiety and hopelessness in patients with vitiligo on an Iranian population. Health Qual Life Outcomes. 2020;18:20.
3. Kumar R, Prasad D. Melanocytorrhagy and apoptosis in vitiligo: connecting jigsaw pieces. Indian J Dermatol Venereol Leprol. 2012;78:19-23.
4. Le Poole IC, Das PK, Van den Wijngaard RM, Bos JD, Westerhof W. Review of etiopathomechanism of vitiligo: a convergence theory. Exp Dermatol. 1993;2:145-53.
5. Migayron L, Boniface K, Seneschal J. Vitiligo, From Physiopathology to Emerging Treatments: A Review. Dermatol Ther (Heidelb). 2020;10(6):1185-98.
6. Rashighi M, Agarwal P, Richmond JM, Harris TH, Dresser K, Su MW, et al. CXCL10 Is Critical for the Progression and Maintenance of Depigmentation in a Mouse Model of Vitiligo. Sci Transl Med. 2014;6(223):223ra23.
7. Nan Y, Wu C, Zhang YJ. Interplay Between Janus Kinase/Signal Transducer and Activator of Transcription Signaling Activated by Type I Interferons and Viral Antagonism. Front Immunol. 2017;8:1758.
8. Yang L, Yang S, Lei J, Hu W, Chen R, Lin F, et al. Role of chemokines and the corresponding receptors in vitiligo: a pilot study. J Dermatol. 2018;45:31-8.
9. Chen X, Guo W, Chang Y, Chen J, Kang P, Yi X, et al. Oxidative Stress- Induced IL-15 Trans-Presentation in Keratinocytes Contributes to CD8(+) T Cells Activation via JAK-STAT Pathway in Vitiligo. Free Radic Biol Med. 2019;139:80-91.
10. O'Shea JJ, Schwartz DM, Villarino AV, Gadina M, McInnes IB, Laurence A. The JAK-STAT Pathway: Impact on Human Disease and Therapeutic Intervention. Annu Rev Med. 2015;66:311-28.
11. Boukhedouni N, Martins C, Darrigade AS, Drullion C, Rambert J, Barrault C, et al. Type-1 Cytokines Regulate MMP-9 Production and E-Cadherin Disruption to Promote Melanocyte Loss in Vitiligo. JCI Insight. 2020;5(11):e133772.
12. Sardana K, Muddebihal A, Khurana A. JAK inhibitors in vitiligo: what they hit and what they miss—an immunopathogenesis based exposition of existing evidence. Expert Rev Clin Pharmacol. 2023;16(12):1221-7.
13. Abduelmula A, Mufti A, Chong DH, Sood S, Sachdeva M, Yeung J. Management of vitiligo with topical janus tyrosine kinase inhibitor therapy: An evidence-based review. JAAD Int. 2022;9: 156-8.
14. Persaud I, Diamond S, Pan R, Burke K, Harris J, Conlin M, et al. Plasma Pharmacokinetics and Distribution of RuxolitinibInto Skin Following Oral and Topical Administration in Minipigs. Int J Pharm. 2020;590:119889.
15. Rosmarin D, Passeron T, Pandya AG, Grimes P, Harris JE, Desai SR, et al.; TRuE-V Study Group. Two Phase 3, Randomized, Controlled Trials of Ruxolitinib Cream for Vitiligo. N Engl J Med. 2022;387(16):1445-55.
16. Sheikh A, Rafique W, Owais R, Malik F, Ali E. FDA approves Ruxolitinib (Opzelura) for Vitiligo Therapy: A breakthrough in the field of dermatology. Ann Med Surg (Lond). 2022;81:104499.
17. Rosmarin D, Pandya AG, Lebwohl M, Grimes P, Hamzavi I, Gottlieb AB, et al. Ruxolitinib Cream for Treatment of Vitiligo: A Randomised, Controlled, Phase 2 Trial. Lancet. 2020;396(10244):110-20.
18. Joshipura D, Plotnikova N, Goldminz A, Deverapalli S, Turkowski Y, Gottlieb A, et al. Importance of light in the treatment of vitiligo with JAK-inhibitors. J Dermatolog Treat. 2018;29(1):98-9.
19. Mobasher P, Guerra R, Li SJ, Frangos J, Ganesan AK, Huang V. Open-label pilot study of tofacitinib 2% for the treatment of refractory vitiligo. Br J Dermatol. 2020;182(4):1047-9.
20. Yagi K, Ishida Y, Otsuka A, Kabashima K. Two cases of vitiligo vulgaris treated with topical Janus kinase inhibitor delgocitinib. Australas J Dermatol. 2021;62(3):433-4.
21. Qi F, Liu F, Gao L. Janus Kinase Inhibitors in the Treatment of Vitiligo: A Review. Front Immunol. 2021;12:790125.
22. Craiglow BG, King BA. Tofacitinib Citrate for the Treatment of Vitiligo: A Pathogenesis-Directed Therapy. JAMA Dermatol. 2015;151(10):1110-2.

23. Liu LY, Strassner JP, Refat MA, Harris JE, King BA. Repigmentation in vitiligo using the Janus kinase inhibitor tofacitinib may require concomitant light exposure. J Am Acad Dermatol. 2017;77(4):675-682.e1.
24. Song H, Hu Z, Zhang S, Yang L, Liu Y, Wang T. Effectiveness and safety of tofacitinib combined with narrowband ultraviolet B phototherapy for patients with refractory vitiligo in real-world clinical practice. Dermatol Ther. 2022;35(11):e15821.
25. Fang WC, Chiu SH, Lin SY, Huang SM, Lan CE. Evaluation of low-dose tofacitinib combining narrowband UVB therapy for treating vitiligo patients who had failed previous therapy: A pilot study. Photodermatol Photoimmunol Photomed. 2021;37(4):345-7.
26. Komnitski M, Komnitski A, Komnitski Junior A, Silva de Castro CC. Partial repigmentation of vitiligo with tofacitinib, without exposure to ultraviolet radiation. An Bras Dermatol. 2020;95(4):473-6.
27. Aickara DJ, Patel S, Rosen J, Alonso-Llamazares J. Significant improvement of vitiligo with oral tofacitinib treatment. Int J Dermatol. 2023;62(6):e358-e360.
28. Harris JE, Rashighi M, Nguyen N, Jabbari A, Ulerio G, Clynes R, et al. Rapid skin repigmentation on oral ruxolitinib in a patient with coexistent vitiligo and alopecia areata (AA). J Am Acad Dermatol. 2016;74(2):370-1.
29. Mumford BP, Gibson A, Chong AH. Repigmentation of vitiligo with oral baricitinib. Australas J Dermatol. 2020;61(4):374-6.
30. Ezzedine K, Peeva E, Yamaguchi Y, Cox LA, Banerjee A, Han G, et al. Efficacy and safety of oral ritlecitinib for the treatment of active nonsegmental vitiligo: A randomized phase 2b clinical trial. J Am Acad Dermatol. 2023;88(2):395-403.
31. Gianfaldoni S, Tchernev G, Wollina U, Roccia MG, Fioranelli M, Lotti J, et al. Micro - Focused Phototherapy Associated To Janus Kinase Inhibitor: A Promising Valid Therapeutic Option for Patients with Localized Vitiligo. Open Access Maced J Med Sci. 2018;6(1):46-8.

CHAPTER 8

JAK Inhibitors for Eczematous Conditions

Soumya Jagadeesan, Prasanna Duraisamy

"Dear Eczema, let's break up."
—Samantha Loya

Overview

- Introduction
- Atopic Dermatitis
- Prurigo Nodularis
- Chronic Actinic Dermatitis
- Allergic Contact Dermatitis
- Expert Opinion

■ INTRODUCTION

Recent advances in molecular targeted treatments are revolutionizing dermatologic therapy. The Janus kinase-signal transducer and activator of transcription (JAK-STAT) pathway is an intracellular signaling pathway that is a critical junction for several different proinflammatory signaling cascades (see Chapter 2). Cytokines and other inflammatory mediators that drive many of the common inflammatory dermatoses depend on JAK-STAT signaling and the inhibition of this pathway using JAK inhibitors can be an effective treatment strategy for these diseases. Over the past decade, JAK inhibitors have been used off-label for multiple dermatological conditions including vitiligo, alopecia areata, psoriasis, and atopic dermatitis (AD). The recent Food and Drug Administration (FDA) approvals for topical JAK inhibitor, ruxolitinib in 2021, and systemic agents, abrocitinib and upadacitinib in 2022, for AD reflect the broadening application of JAK inhibitors in dermatology.[1] This chapter discusses the application of JAK inhibitors in managing AD and other eczematous disorders.

■ ATOPIC DERMATITIS

Atopic dermatitis has a complex pathogenesis involving genetic and environmental factors, defects in the epidermal barrier, and immune dysregulation. In AD, the impairment of the epidermal barrier is caused by reduced production of key elements like filaggrin, tight junctions, fatty acids, and ceramides. Furthermore, there is an imbalance in the skin surface microbiome, notably increased staphylococcal colonization. These factors facilitate enhanced transepidermal penetration of allergens, thereby inciting skin inflammation. Activated Langerhans cells and keratinocytes release alarmins including interleukin 25 (IL-25), IL-33, and thymic stromal lymphopoietin (TSLP), which serve as key drivers of the inflammatory process in AD.[1,2]

The immunopathogenesis of AD is a predominant Th2-mediated immune response with additional T helper 22 (Th22), and Th17-driven inflammation in the acute stages and an increasing role of Th1 in the chronic lesions. In the acute phase, stimulation by triggers causes release of Th2 cytokines—IL-4, IL-5, IL-13, and IL-31. IL-4 and IL-13, the key effector cytokines of AD, activate and promote proliferation of Th2 cells, activation of dendritic and myeloid cells, and induction of immunoglobulin E (IgE) class-switching in B cells. IL-5 is involved in the activation, differentiation, and migration of eosinophils. IL-4, IL-13, IL-31, and IL-33 also increase skin barrier impairment by reducing the expression of epidermal proteins, such as filaggrin, loricrin, and involucrin in both lesional and nonlesional skin. IL-31, TSLP, substance P, and IL-4 act as pruritogens and the resultant scratching further increases the epidermal barrier damage and inflammation. In the chronic stage of AD, there is a role of Th1-mediated immune response characterized by increased IL-12, interferon gamma (IFN-γ), and granulocyte-macrophage colony-stimulating factor (GM-CSF). These induce keratinocyte apoptosis and additional inflammation in the skin, leading to a sustained itch-scratch cycle and lichenification.[2]

Role of Cytokines in Atopic Dermatitis and Why Janus Kinase Inhibitors Work?

Interleukin-4 and Interleukin-13

Interleukin-4 acts through the IL-4 receptor (IL-4R) complex, which has two subtypes—type I IL-4R composed of IL-4R alpha (IL-4Rα) chain and a common gamma chain and type II IL-4R comprising an IL-4Rα chain and an IL-13R alpha-1 (IL-13Rα1) chain. Due to the presence of the IL-13Rα1 chain, IL-13 can also exert effects by binding to type II IL-4R. Different JAKs are bound to the different receptor subunits and for the IL4R class—JAK1, JAK3, and tyrosine kinase 2 (TYK2) are bound to IL-4Rα, γc chain, and IL-13Rα, respectively.[2] This via STAT3 and STAT6 and leads to Th2 cell differentiation, B-cell proliferation, and IgE class-switching. The effector cytokines released are IL-5, IL-10, and IL-13, which further activate inflammation.[3]

Interleukin-31

The IL-31R is made of an IL-31R alpha (IL-31Rα) chain and an oncostatin M receptor beta chain. IL-31 binding activates JAK1 and JAK2, stimulating STAT3, STAT5, and, to a lesser extent, STAT1. This also activates eosinophils, Th2 cells, and further secretion of IL-4 and IL-13. IL-31 is also a key itch mediator.[2,3]

Thymic Stromal Lymphopoietin

Thymic stromal lymphopoietin is produced by keratinocytes and acts on group 2 innate lymphoid cells (ILC2) and dendritic cells. It binds to a receptor comprised IL-7R alpha (IL-7Rα) and TSLP receptors and phosphorylates JAK1 and JAK2, activating STAT5. It induces dendritic cell activation and migration along with Th2-cell differentiation to release IL-4, IL-5, and IL-13. TSLP may help sustain the itch-scratch cycle in AD as mechanical injury increases TSLP expression, which again increases the Th2 responses. TSLP also increases the secretion of periostin through the JAK/STAT pathway, which triggers histamine-independent itch.[1,2]

Interleukin-22

Interleukin-22 is produced by Th22 cells and plays increasing role in the chronic stages of the disease. It acts via JAK1 and TYK2 and causes keratinocyte proliferation and epidermal thickening. It also inhibits differentiation and reduces production of barrier function proteins, contributing to lichenification.[1,2]

Considering that the multiple inflammatory cytokines involved in the pathology of AD all function through the JAK-STAT pathway, especially JAK1, inhibiting JAK-STAT pathway is a logical treatment strategy as it can simultaneously disrupt multiple cytokines at different areas of the inflammatory cascade.

Systemic Janus Kinase Inhibitors

Varied JAK inhibitors have been used and approved in AD and are discussed in detail in Chapter 5 and a brief summary is given here.

Upadacitinib: It is a selective JAK1 inhibitor and is approved by the FDA for treatment of refractory, moderate-to-severe AD in adults and children ≥12 years of age. The dose varies from 15 to 30 mg with a better response in the higher dose.[1,2] There is rapid onset of action with lesional clearance as early as week 2 and pruritus relief as early as week 1. Upadacitinib was found to have superior efficacy over dupilumab, producing faster disease clearance and itch relief in the early time points of the study.[4]

Abrocitinib: This selective JAK1 inhibitor approved by the United States FDA (USFDA) and launched in India has a dose of 100–200 mg. Reduction of dose to 50 mg is warranted for patients with renal impairment, patients on cytochrome P450-2C19 inhibitors, and patients who have reduced activity of cytochrome P450-2C19.[1,2] A higher dose has a better response and is superior to dupilumab in the early treatment phases, with the response becoming similar in the later stages. Abrocitinib has also shown efficacy in dupilumab nonresponders.[4] Increased incidence of nausea was noted with abrocitinib (≤15%) versus upadacitinib (≤3%) while acne occurred at lesser rates—abrocitinib (≤5%) versus upadacitinib (≤17%). Transient dose-dependent reduction in platelet counts was noted with maximum reduction at week 4 of treatment followed by recovery to baseline.[1,2]

Baricitinib: It is an oral JAK1/JAK2 selective inhibitor and was approved in Europe (October 2020) for moderate-to-severe AD and a dose of 4 mg daily is effective (**Figs. 1 and 2**) with a reduced doses of 2 mg have been used in patients with renal impairment.[1,2] The most common serious infection was eczema herpeticum. Baricitinib causes slight increase in platelet counts and minimal changes in other hematologic parameters.[1,2]

Tofacitinib: It is a pan-JAK inhibitor with a primary affinity for JAK1 and JAK3 and lesser affinity with JAK2 and TYK2. Its use in AD is off-label.[1,2] In a study of six patients with moderate-to-severe refractory AD, significant clinical improvements was observed with oral tofacitinib, with five receiving 5 mg twice daily and one receiving 5 mg once daily [66.6% reduction in the SCORAD (SCORing Atopic Dermatitis)].[2] In our experience with tofacitinib in AD, we noted a rapid reduction in the lesions—clear/almost clear at the end of 1 month of treatment which was maintained on follow-up,[5] which was maintained on follow-up. It has also been used in baricitinib refractory AD and as a rescue therapy with dupilumab.[6,7] While we have seen its superlative results as the drug is off patent and affordable, we hope that more data is generated on its use in AD.

Topical Janus Kinase Inhibitors

Since the measured plasma levels seen with topical JAK inhibitors are less than the lower limit needed for systemic inhibition, topical JAK inhibitors can be an alternative that can provide local effects without any systemic risks.[3,8]

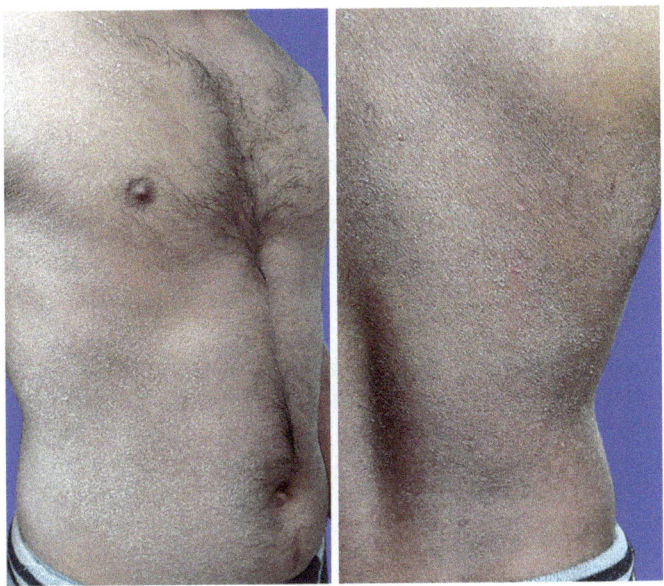

FIG. 1: Atopic dermatitis in an 18-year-old boy with repeated relapses and history of erythroderma, and poor control despite administering cyclosporine.

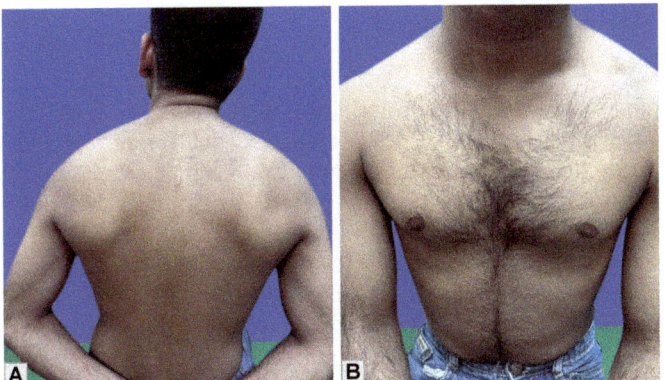

FIGS. 2A AND B: Good response to baricitinib 4 mg OD after 2 weeks. He is asymptomatic on baricitinib 4 mg.
Courtesy: Professor GK Singh.

Ruxolitinib: This selective inhibitor of JAK1 and JAK2 is available as a 1.5% cream formulation and is approved for the short-term or intermittent treatment of mild-to-moderate AD in patients 12 years and older. Notably, when compared to topical triamcinolone, topical ruxolitinib showed similar reduction in the Eczema Area and Severity Index (EASI) scores, but most cases of AD need a higher potency steroid; hence, the efficacy of this drug in refractory cases may not be promising. Application should not exceed 60 g (1 tube) per week or 100 g per 2 weeks.[3,8]

Tofacitinib: Topical tofacitinib is available as 2% ointment and gel formulations. In a vehicle-controlled trial, topical tofacitinib 2% twice daily showed rapid results during the first week, which was sustained over a 4-week treatment course. Improvements in Itch Severity Index scores were noted after 1 week of treatment. Adverse events noted were mild to moderate such as nasopharyngitis, headaches, and bronchitis.[3,8]

Delgocitinib: It is a pan-JAK inhibitor and is approved in Japan for treating AD in adults (0.5% ointment) and children (0.25%). It has achieved reasonable results and is being investigated as a potential treatment option for chronic hand eczema. In animal models, it was also found to improve the skin barrier function by increasing production of filaggrin and other barrier factors.[3,8]

Summary

Rapid onset of action is one of the key advantages with JAK inhibitors, especially with regard to control of pruritus apart from the fact that they have a short half-life. They can be useful for patients who require a rapid response, can be used as intermittent treatment in patients with seasonal flares. However, JAK inhibitors are associated with wider range of adverse effects and have to be restricted for at-risk populations. Although studies in AD have shown a favorable safety profile, there are still potential safety concerns[1,9] (see Chapter 11).

■ PRURIGO NODULARIS

Prurigo nodularis (PN) is a chronic inflammatory disorder characterized by intensely pruritic, hyperkeratotic nodules over the trunk and the extremities.[10]

Pathogenesis

Although not fully understood, the underlying pathophysiology of PN is thought to be a neuroimmune dysregulation leading to a persistent "itch scratch" vicious cycle, leading to recurrent skin excoriation and nodule. There is aberrant dermal and epidermal nerve fiber density. Neuroinflammation mediated by neurotrophins and neuropeptides like substance P and calcitonin gene-related peptide along with keratinocyte signaling lead to a Th2-mediated immune response with key cytokine mediators IL-31, IL-4, and oncostatin M, which mediate their action via the JAK-STAT pathway. There is also evidence of role of other molecules like IL-13, IL-17, IL-22, and TSLP in PN lesions that can increase inflammation and release of pruritogens. Immunostaining has shown increased expression of STAT3 and STAT6 in lesional skin in PN favoring the role of multiple cytokine pathways, such as Th2, Th17, and Th22.[11]

Why Janus Kinase Inhibitors?

Considering the role of multiple cytokines from the Th2, Th17, and Th22 pathways and STAT1/3/6 upregulation in PN, a JAK inhibitor that can work across multiple cytokines would be ideal for treating PN.[11]

To date, tofacitinib, baricitinib, and upadacitinib have been used successfully to treat PN in small case series and case reports (Table 1), and an expert panel consensus on PN recommends JAK inhibitors when all other options are exhausted.[10] It has been compared with dupilumab and patients on JAK-inhibitors had a faster first response than those on dupilumab.[12]

TABLE 1	A summary of salient data on JAK inhibitor in prurigo nodularis.			
Authors	Drug	Dose	Outcome	Adverse event
Liu et al., 9 patients[13]	Tofacitinib	5 mg twice daily	Complete resolution of itch in 100% at 1 week. 77.78% had complete clearance of lesions at 6 months	Nil
Sardana et al., 1 patient[11]	Tofacitinib	5 mg twice daily 4 weeks then once daily for 2 months	Resolution of itch and sleep disturbances in 10 days	Nil
Muntaner-Virgili et al., 1 patient[14]	Upadacitinib	15 mg twice a day	Complete clearance of lesions and itch at week 16	Nil
Duraisamy et al., 1 patient[5]	Tofacitinib	5 mg twice a day	PGA 0 at 1 month of treatment with sustained response at 3 months	Weight gain
Yin et al., 1 patient	Baricitinib	4 mg once a day	Marked improvement in pruritus in 1 week. Near-complete clearance at 4 months	Nil

(JAK: Janus kinase; PGA: physician global assessment)

Source: Yin M. Dermatol Ther. 2022;35:E15642.

■ CHRONIC ACTINIC DERMATITIS

Chronic actinic dermatitis (CAD) is a photosensitive disorder caused by chronic and pruritic eczematous lesions on sun-exposed areas. The underlying pathogenetic mechanisms of CAD are not exactly known, but a T-cell mediated immune response to an ultraviolet (UV)-induced autoantigen or a contact allergy to exogenous allergens may be involved. A recent study on the photoimmunopathogenesis of CAD noted an altered immune response with an increase in certain T-cell types (CD4+, CD8+, IL-17+, IFN-γ+, and common-γ chain receptor+ cells).[15] Since common-γ chain receptors and other specific cytokine receptors work through downstream JAK1/JAK3 signaling, JAK inhibitors may have a role in the management of CAD. Multiple reports have described use of tofacitinib,[5,16] baricitinib, upadacitinib and abrocitinib (Table 2).[17,18]

■ ALLERGIC CONTACT DERMATITIS

Allergic contact dermatitis (ACD) is a type IV delayed-type hypersensitivity reaction, involving two main phases: Sensitization and elicitation. During sensitization, a foreign substance penetrates the skin and activates innate immunity mediated by cytokines like IL-1α, IL-1β, and tumor necrosis factor alpha (TNF-α). Allergens captured by antigen-presenting cells (APCs) then migrate to lymph nodes, activating specific T cells (Th1, Th2, Th17, and Treg), which then differentiate as effector and memory cells. Upon re-exposure, the hapten-specific T-cells recognize the allergen, triggering an inflammatory response mediated by cytokines like IFN-γ, IL-2, IL-12, and IL-17, leading to the clinical symptoms of ACD.[19] Recent studies highlight hapten specificity in the T-cell immune responses: Nickel primarily activates Th1 and Th17 pathways, while substances like rubber and fragrances trigger Th2 pathways. Since the JAK-STAT signaling is involved in the downstream cascade of these cytokines and also in pruritis pathways, JAK inhibitor is a promising therapeutic option for ACD.[20]

TABLE 2	Overview of JAK inhibitor in CAD.			
Authors	Drug	Dose	Outcome	Adverse event
Majid et al.*	Tofacitinib	5 mg twice a day, tapered to once daily after 6 months	Clearing of lesions within 4–8 weeks of initiation of therapy	Nil
Vesely et al.*	Tofacitinib	5 mg twice a day	Clearing of lesions within 8 weeks of initiation of therapy	Herpes zoster
Dev et al.[16]	Tofacitinib	5 mg twice a day	Significant response at 6 weeks, near-complete clearance at 3 months	Nil
Duraisamy et al.[5]	Tofacitinib	5 mg twice a day	PGA 0 at 1 months of treatment	Perianal abscess
Jin et al.*	Abrocitinib	100 mg once a day	Significant improvement at 6 weeks	Nil
Maguire et al.*	Baricitinib	2 mg once a day	EASI of 0.5 at 9 months. Complete clearance at 16 months	Blisters over fingers

*Majid I. Dermatol Ther. 2022;35:e15467; Vesely MD. JAAD Case Rep. 2017;3:4-6; Jin X, Qiao J. Am J Ther. 23, Maguire J. Skin Health Dis. 2023;3(6):e243.

(CAD: chronic actinic dermatitis; EASI: Eczema Area and Severity Index; JAK: Janus kinase; PGA: physician global assessment)

The varied disorders that have shown exquisite response to JAK inhibitors range from **compositae airborne dermatitis** with response to abrocitinib[21] and tofacitinib.[22] The authors have also successfully used tofacitinib 5 mg twice daily in patients of **ACD** unresponsive to conventional immunosuppressants.[5]

Another emerging indication is **chronic hand eczema**, where the cytokine milieu is Th2 based and is amenable to JAK inhibitor across phenotypes.[23]

■ EXPERT OPINION

Janus kinase inhibitors represent a significant advancement in dermatologic therapy, offering a promising treatment for various eczematous dermatoses like AD, PN, CAD, and ACD. They have been shown to provide rapid symptom relief, especially with regard to pruritus. There is a need for studies on their long-term safety and their use must be balanced against potential adverse effects. Careful patient selection and monitoring is essential when choosing JAK inhibitors as a treatment option.

■ REFERENCES

1. Munera-Campos M, Carrascosa JM. Janus Kinase Inhibitors in Atopic Dermatitis: New Perspectives. Actas Dermosifiliogr. 2023;114(8):680-707.
2. Mikhaylov D, Ungar B, Renert-Yuval Y, Guttman-Yassky E. Oral Janus kinase inhibitors for atopic dermatitis. Ann Allergy Asthma Immunol. 2023;130(5):577-92.
3. Nakashima C, Yanagihara S, Otsuka A. Innovation in the treatment of atopic dermatitis: Emerging topical and oral Janus kinase inhibitors. Allergol Int. 2022;71(1):40-6.
4. Gao Q, Zhao Y, Zhang J. Efficacy and safety of abrocitinib and upadacitinib versus dupilumab in adults with moderate-to-severe atopic dermatitis: A systematic review and meta-analysis. Heliyon. 2023;9(6):e16704.

5. Duraisamy P, Jagadeesan S, Thomas J. Tofacitinib in the treatment of refractory eczemas - a case series. J Dermatol Treat. 2022;33(6):2873-5.
6. Dhir B, Meena SK, Sardana K, Sharath S. Use of tofacitinib in baricitinib-refractory atopic dermatitis: An example of JAK inhibitor switching. Pediatr Dermatol. 2024;41(1):139-40.
7. Peterson DM, Vesely MD. Remission of severe atopic dermatitis with dupilumab and rescue tofacitinib therapy. JAAD Case Reports. 2021;10:4-7.
8. Fardos MI, Singh R, Perche PO, Kelly KA, Feldman SR. Evaluating topical JAK inhibitors as a treatment option for atopic dermatitis. Expert Rev Clin Immunol. 2022;18(3):221-31.
9. Yoon S, Kim K, Shin K, Kim HS, Kim B, Kim MB, et al. The safety of systemic Janus kinase inhibitors in atopic dermatitis: A systematic review and meta-analysis of randomized controlled trials. J Eur Acad Dermatol Venereol. 2024;38(1):52-61.
10. Elmariah S, Kim B, Berger T, Chisolm S, Kwatra SG, Mollanazar N, et al. Practical approaches for diagnosis and management of prurigo nodularis: United States expert panel consensus. J Am Acad Dermatol. 2021;84(3):747-60.
11. Sardana K, Rose Mathachan S, Agrawal D. Treatment of recalcitrant paediatric prurigo nodularis with tofacitinib, an exquisite example of bench-to-bedside translation of JAK-STAT expression. Indian J Dermatol Venereol Leprol. 2023:1-3.
12. Yew YW, Yeo PM. Comparison between dupilumab and oral Janus kinase inhibitors in the treatment of prurigo nodularis with or without atopic dermatitis in a tertiary care center in Singapore. JAAD Int. 2023;13:13-4.
13. Liu T, Chu Y, Wang Y, Zhong X, Yang C, Bai J, et al. Successful treatment of prurigo nodularis with tofacitinib: The experience from a single center. Int J Dermatol. 2023;62(5):e293-5.
14. Muntaner-Virgili C, Moreno-Vilchez C, Torrecilla-Vall-Llossera C, Figueras-Nart I. Upadacitinib for prurigo nodularis: A case report. JAAD Case Reports. 2023;S235251262300070X.
15. Kim JH, Kim HJ, Yoo DW, Park KD, Kwon HJ, Seo JW, et al. A postulated model for photoimmunopathogenesis of chronic actinic dermatitis around adaptive immunity, including Th17 cells, Tregs, TRMs, cytotoxic T cells, and/or common-γ chain receptor+ cells. Photodermatol Photoimmunol Photomed. 2023;39(2):147-54.
16. Dev A, Bishnoi A, Narang T, Vinay K. Recalcitrant chronic actinic dermatitis responding to tofacitinib: A case report. IJDVL. 2023;89(4):600-2.
17. Jin X, Qiao J. Effectiveness of Abrocitinib in a Patient With Chronic Actinic Dermatitis. Am J Ther. 2022. [Online ahead of print]
18. Pappa G, Sgouros D, Kanelleas A, Koumaki D, Bozi E, Katoulis A. JAK-ing up chronic actinic dermatitis with upadacitinib. Clin Exp Dermatol. 2023;49(2):173-5.
19. Tramontana M, Hansel K, Bianchi L, Sensini C, Malatesta N, Stingeni L. Advancing the understanding of allergic contact dermatitis: from pathophysiology to novel therapeutic approaches. Front Med. 2023;10:1184289.
20. Johnson H, Guenther J, Adler BL, Yu J. Janus Kinase Inhibitors: A Promising Therapeutic Option for Allergic Contact Dermatitis. Cutis. 2023;111(2):92-105.
21. Baltazar D, Shinamoto SR, Hamann CP, Hamann D, Hamann CR. Occupational airborne allergic contact dermatitis to invasive Compositae species treated with abrocitinib: a case report. Contact Dermatitis. 2022;87(6):542-4.
22. Muddebihal A, Sardana K, Sinha S, Kumar D. Tofacitinib in refractory Parthenium-induced airborne allergic contact dermatitis. Contact Dermatitis. 2023;88(2):150-2.
23. Zalewski A, Szepietowski JC. Topical and systemic JAK inhibitors in hand eczema - a narrative review. Expert Rev Clin Immunol. 2023;19(4):365-73.

CHAPTER 9

JAK Inhibitors in Pruritic Disorders

Ramkumar Ramamoorthy, Kabir Sardana

"Nothing is more powerful than an idea whose time has come."
—Victor Hugo

Overview
- Introduction
- Rationale of Janus Kinase inhibitors

■ INTRODUCTION

Itch is a prominent and distressing symptom in many dermatological disorders. Pruritus is a cardinal feature of atopic dermatitis (AD)[1] and lichen planus (LP).[2] Around 70% of patients diagnosed with psoriasis report itch in involved and uninvolved skin as well.[2] Therefore, any medication which gives adequate relief from this uncomfortable sensation is always a welcome addition to a therapeutic armamentarium for the treatment of skin diseases in routine practice.

In this section we provide a summary of the promising results shown by Janus kinase inhibitors (JAKis) in providing itch relief in skin disorders and discuss the scope for using a JAKi in managing itch in various skin disorders in the near future.

■ RATIONALE OF JANUS KINASE INHIBITORS

Janus kinase-signal transducer and activator of transcription (JAK-STAT) pathway is the major pathway employed by cytokines for intracellular signal transduction besides other pathways activated in various cell types.[3]

One of these signaling cascades is mediated by JAKs (also see Chapter 2). Recently, it could be shown on a molecular level that JAK1 directly activates frontal cortex neurons and thus can cause chronic itching.[4] This was revealed by knock down experiments conducted in mouse, which suggested a key role for JAK1, a ubiquitously expressed enzyme in human body in mediating itch signaling through sensory neurons, and therefore play a significant role in inducing neurogenic inflammation in skin diseases.

Several cytokines act on receptors present in sensory neurons to mediate itch[1] either directly [interleukin 31 (IL-31), thymic stromal lymphopoietin (TSLP), IL-2, and IL-17] or indirectly by sensitizing the neurons to other cytokines (IL-4 by lowering the threshold for response to histamine and IL-31). Itch is mainly transmitted through unmyelinated type C

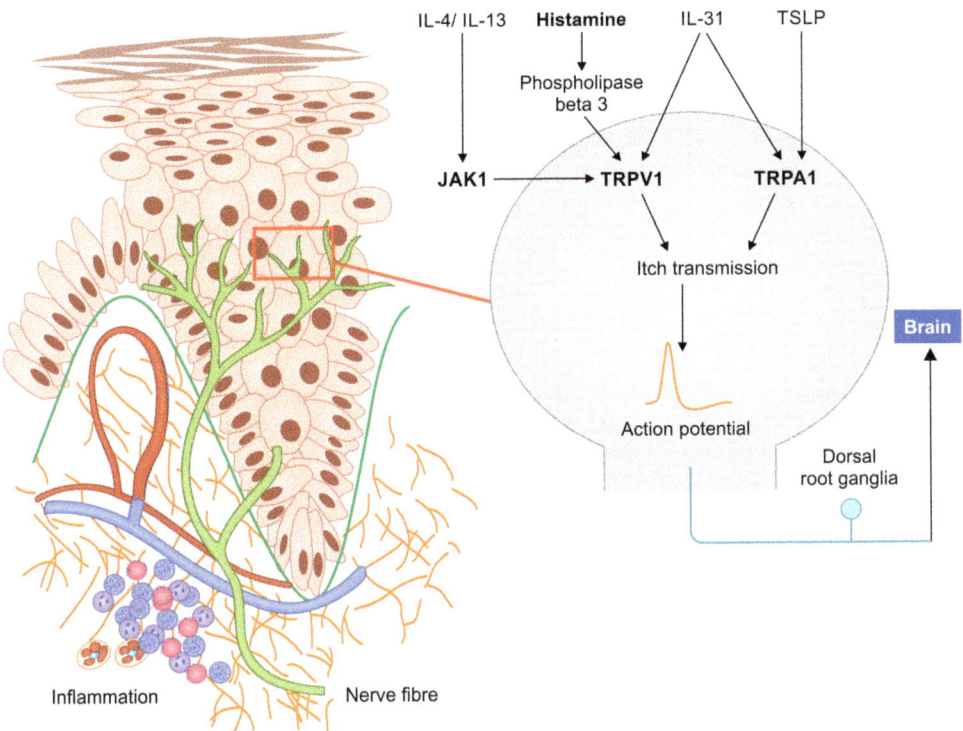

(IL: interleukin; JAK1: Janus kinase 1; TSLP: thymic stromal lymphopoietin; TRPA1: transient receptor potential ankyrin 1; TRPV1: transient receptor potential vanilloid 1)

FIG. 1: Overview of the role of JAK1 receptor and cytokines and their role in transmission of the sensation of itch.

fibers in dermoepidermal junction and epidermis by several mediators with a key role for TRPV channels [transient receptor potential vanilloid 1 and ankyrin 1 (TRPV1 and TRPA1)] in the signaling cascade (**Fig. 1**). Among the list of mediators, proteases such as tryptase released from mast cell and serine esterases from epidermis signal through protease-activated receptors (PARs), which play a major role in transmitting nonhistaminergic itch. PAR-2 receptors have been shown to activate TRPV channels through protein kinase C-dependent signaling pathway.[5] Thus, T helper 2 (Th2) immunity is a driver of chronic pruritus and these cell lines are active in AD and in other Th2-dominated inflammatory and pruritic skin disorders (**Box 1**). IL-4, IL-13, and IL-31 are not only proinflammatory mediators but are strong pruritogenic cytokines.

Atopic Dermatitis—Effect of Janus Kinase inhibitors in Itch Relief

The itch relief in AD patients on treatment with JAKis is dramatic and sustained until the end of study period in the published studies where the itch severity is documented by employing universally validated scoring systems. Rapid relief from pruritus was noted within days of instituting treatment. Earliest improvement was observed within 24 hours after intake of abrocitinib,[6] 1 week for 4 mg of baricitinib,[8] and 2 week after intake of 2 mg of baricitinib. Upadacitinib relieved itch within 2 days of the initial dose of treatment.[7] More than 4 points improvement in the Numerical Rating Scale (NRS) score [Peak Pruritus (PP)-NRS 4] was observed after 2 weeks of therapy with 30 mg upadacitinib per day and with

> **BOX 1** T helper 2 (Th2)-mediated skin disorders.
>
> - Atopic dermatitis
> - Bullous pemphigoid
> - Chronic pruritus of unknown origin (CPUO)
> - Cutaneous helminth infestations
> - Cutaneous T-cell lymphoma
> - Insect bite reactions
> - Prurigo nodularis
> - Scabies

200 mg abrocitinib. Similar improvement was noted after 6 weeks of treatment with 4 mg of baricitinib. Overall upadacitinib 30 mg is ranked as the most efficacious medication for AD and is the most potent inhibitor JAK1 in cellular assays, which corresponds to the itch relief.[8,9]

In AD, abrocitinib[10,11] via its action on JAK1 and JAK2 can block the cytokines IL-31, TSLP via its inhibition of common gamma chain cytokines. Abrocitinib (200 mg) was found to be better in itch relief than dupilumab[12,13] due to inhibition of multiple cytokines which signal through JAK-STAT pathway. Notably, this superiority was not noted for 100 mg of abrocitinb[14] and has been explained by the less pronounced action of abrocitinib on JAK2 enzyme, which mediates signal transduction from IL-5.[15]

Similarly, 30 mg daily of upadacitinib achieved faster and superior itch control than dupilumab during 16 weeks of treatment in adults with moderate to severe AD[16] and was also superior to baricitinib and/or dupilumab.[17]

The other drugs that have been trialed in AD include baricitinib,[18] ruxolitinib (1.5%),[19] tofacitinib (1–3%),[20,21] while delgocitinib (a pan JAKi) has been used both in AD and hand eczema.[22]

While tofacitinib was developed to target JAK3, it also targets JAK1 and JAK2 and tends to work on multiple cytokines of the Th1, Th2, and Th17 family, even though it is the least potent inhibitor of interferon alpha signaling among all JAKis.[8] However, barring few case reports, published studies done on oral tofacitinib usage in AD are not available,[23,24] even though in real world settings the drug tends to work in moderate to severe AD (see Chapters 5 and 8).

Psoriasis—Itch Relief from Janus Kinase Inhibitors

Itch in psoriatic patients is attributed to the release of several mediators, such as neuropeptides, opioids, vascular endothelial growth factor, and some cytokines such as IL-2, IL-31, and IL-17A.[25] Nerve growth factor is known to upregulate the activity of transient receptor potential (TRP) channels. Oral tofacitinib 10 mg twice a day was shown to be noninferior to etanercept.[26] Also topical tofacitinib improved itch score by 4 weeks of routine use.[27] Tofacitinib gave relief from pruritus in both 10 and 20 mg daily doses. Deucravacitinib, a JAKi, which selectively inhibits pseudokinase domain of tyrosine kinase 2 (TYK2), has also been found to efficacious in psoriasis with a sustained improvement till 52 weeks. The itch control was significant for the skin and scalp lesions.[28]

Lichen Planus—Itch Relief from Janus Kinase Inhibitors

Itch in LP is not a well-studied subject. Several cytokines[29,30] released by multiple polarized T-cell subsets have been implicated including IL-31, IL-5, IL-10, IL-17, tumor necrosis factor alpha (TNF-α) in addition to mast cell-derived tryptase and serine protease produced by epidermis, which mediate pruritus through PARs type 2 in sensory neurons. Upregulation of TRPV1 channels has been reported in mucosal LP.[31]

Tofacitinib 10 mg/day has been found to give satisfactory results in few cases.[32] More studies are needed to explore the possibility of using topical and systemic JAKis to manage pruritus in LP patients.

Prurigo Nodularis

The itch in prurigo nodularis is mediated by Th2 signaling, resulting in high levels of expression of IL-31, IL-13, and IL-4. Other factors that are implicated include matrix metalloproteinases, insulin-like growth factors, periostin, neurotrophic factors, and CXCL2.[33,34] Upregulation of TRPV1 channels and a dysregulated Th17 axis also result in excessive expression of IL-23 and IL-17A.[33,35] In an open phase 2 trial a daily oral dose of 200 mg of abrocitinib decreased pruritus scores significantly in 80% of patients who were diagnosed with prurigo nodularis.[36] Recently, reports of sustained and dramatic reduction in lesions have been reported from India (see Chapters 8 and 10).

Chronic Pruritus of Unknown Origin

Chronic pruritus of unknown origin (CPUO) is a distressing disorder, which is characterized by a lack of obvious skin changes with concomitant intense itching with a predominant finding of marked eosinophilia ($> 4\%$ or > 0.30 K/mm^3). Varied agents have been tried including antihistamines, mirtazapine [noradrenergic and specific serotonergic antidepressant (NaSSA)], and gabapentinoids (gabapentin and pregabalin) with no consistently effective treatment regimen. Published data has revealed that Th2 immune pathways and the associated cytokines (IL-4, IL-10, IL-13, and IL-33) mediate itching.[1,2] This is consistent with the concept of "immunosenescence" with loss of Th1 cell-driven protective immunity and skewing toward an allergic Th2 response.[3] Also, IL-4 receptor alpha (IL-4Rα) and JAK1 mediate sensory neuron activation, cause chronic itching (**Fig. 1**). A recent study administered tofacitinib 10 mg with a reduction in itching, which was sustained during the study duration. The rationale is that the signaling of major cytokines in CPUO is via JAK heterodimers (IL-4, JAK1/3; IL-13, JAK1/TYK2; IL-5, JAK1/2; and IL-31, JAK1/2), thus a drug that inhibits JAK1, 2, 3 seemed to be ideal for CPUO.[37]

■ SUMMARY

Immune responses in Th2 immunodermatoses (AD and LP) typically involve a complex interplay of multiple cytokines. JAKis target intracellular pathways shared by multiple cytokines. While JAKis do not continuously or completely inhibit cytokine signaling, they have shown impressive results in relieving itch associated with AD due to their impact on multiple cytokines. Selective JAKis are more effective and act faster than dupilumab in reducing itch severity due to AD. Topical JAKis provide itch relief within days of treatment initiation. Thus, JAK inhibition is emerging as a promising new therapeutic strategy to reduce pruritus in various skin disorders. Upcoming trials will provide more knowledge on the role of JAKis in the management of itch associated with psoriasis and LP.

■ REFERENCES

1. Yosipovitch G, Rosen JD, Hashimoto T. Itch: From mechanism to (novel) therapeutic approaches. J Allergy Clin Immunol. 2018;142(5):1375-90.

2. Welz-Kubiak K, Reich A, Szepietowski JC. Clinical Aspects of Itch in Lichen Planus. Acta Derm Venereol. 2017;97(4):505-8.
3. Hu X, Li J, Fu M, Zhao X, Wang W. The JAK/STAT signaling pathway: from bench to clinic. Signal Transduct Target Ther. 2021;6(1):402.
4. Oetjen LK, Mack MR, Feng J, Whelan TM, Niu H, Guo CJ, et al. Sensory Neurons Co-opt Classical Immune Signaling Pathways to Mediate Chronic Itch. Cell. 2017;171(1):217-228.e13.
5. Amadesi S, Cottrell GS, Divino L, Chapman K, Grady EF, Bautista F, et al. Protease-activated receptor 2 sensitizes TRPV1 by protein kinase Cepsilon- and A-dependent mechanisms in rats and mice. J Physiol. 2006;575(Pt 2):555-71.
6. Silverberg JI, Simpson EL, Thyssen JP, Gooderham M, Chan G, Feeney C, et al. Efficacy and Safety of Abrocitinib in Patients With Moderate-to-Severe Atopic Dermatitis: A Randomized Clinical Trial. JAMA Dermatol. 2020;156(8):863-73.
7. Simpson EL, Papp KA, Blauvelt A, Chu CY, Hong HC, Katoh N, et al. Efficacy and Safety of Upadacitinib in Patients With Moderate to Severe Atopic Dermatitis: Analysis of Follow-up Data From the Measure Up 1 and Measure Up 2 Randomized Clinical Trials. JAMA Dermatol. 2022;158(4):404-13.
8. Taylor PC, Choy E, Baraliakos X, Szekanecz Z, Xavier RM, Isaacs JD, et al. Differential properties of Janus kinase inhibitors in the treatment of immune-mediated inflammatory diseases. Rheumatology (Oxford). 2023;63(2):298-308.
9. Silverberg JI, Hong HC, Thyssen JP, Calimlim BM, Joshi A, Teixeira HD, et al. Comparative Efficacy of Targeted Systemic Therapies for Moderate to Severe Atopic Dermatitis without Topical Corticosteroids: Systematic Review and Network Meta-analysis. Dermatol Ther (Heidelb). 2022;12(5):1181-96.
10. Deeks ED, Duggan S. Abrocitinib: First Approval. Drugs. 2021;81(18):2149-15.
11. Alexis A, de Bruin-Weller M, Weidinger S, Soong W, Barbarot S, Ionita I, et al. Rapidity of Improvement in Signs/Symptoms of Moderate-to-Severe Atopic Dermatitis by Body Region with Abrocitinib in the Phase 3 JADE COMPARE Study. Dermatol Ther (Heidelb). 2022;12(3):771-85.
12. Bieber T, Simpson EL, Silverberg JI, Thaçi D, Paul C, Pink AE, et al.; JADE COMPARE Investigators. Abrocitinib versus Placebo or Dupilumab for Atopic Dermatitis. N Engl J Med. 2021;384(12):1101-12.
13. Shi VY, Bhutani T, Fonacier L, Deleuran M, Shumack S, Valdez H, et al. Phase 3 efficacy and safety of abrocitinib in adults with moderate-to-severe atopic dermatitis after switching from dupilumab (JADE EXTEND). J Am Acad Dermatol. 2022;87(2):351-8.
14. Eichenfield LF, Flohr C, Sidbury R, Siegfried E, Szalai Z, Galus R, et al. Efficacy and Safety of Abrocitinib in Combination With Topical Therapy in Adolescents With Moderate-to-Severe Atopic Dermatitis: The JADE TEEN Randomized Clinical Trial. JAMA Dermatol. 2021;157(10):1165-73.
15. Ogata N, Kouro T, Yamada A, Koike M, Hanai N, Ishikawa T, et al. JAK2 and JAK1 constitutively associate with an IL-5 receptor alpha and betac subunit, respectively, and are activated upon IL-5 stimulation. Blood. 1998;91(7):2264-71.
16. Blauvelt A, Teixeira HD, Simpson EL, Costanzo A, De Bruin-Weller M, Barbarot S, et al. Efficacy and Safety of Upadacitinib vs Dupilumab in Adults With Moderate-to-Severe Atopic Dermatitis: A Randomized Clinical Trial. JAMA Dermatol. 2021;157(9):1047-55.
17. Boesjes CM, Van der Gang LF, Zuithoff NPA, Bakker DS, Spekhorst LS, Haeck I, et al. Effectiveness of Upadacitinib in Patients with Atopic Dermatitis including those with Inadequate Response to Dupilumab and/or Baricitinib: Results from the BioDay Registry. Acta Derm Venereol. 2023;103:adv00872.
18. Radi G, Simonetti O, Rizzetto G, Diotallevi F, Molinelli E, Offidani A. Baricitinib: The First Jak Inhibitor Approved in Europe for the Treatment of Moderate to Severe Atopic Dermatitis in Adult Patients. Healthcare (Basel). 2021;9(11):1575.
19. Papp K, Szepietowski JC, Kircik L, Toth D, Eichenfield LF, Leung DYM, et al. Efficacy and safety of ruxolitinib cream for the treatment of atopic dermatitis: Results from 2 phase 3, randomized, double-blind studies. J Am Acad Dermatol. 2021;85(4):863-72.
20. Bissonnette R, Papp KA, Poulin Y, Gooderham M, Raman M, Mallbris L, et al. Topical tofacitinib for atopic dermatitis: a phase IIa randomized trial. Br J Dermatol. 2016;175(5):902-11.

21. Landis MN, Smith SR, Berstein G, Fetterly G, Ghosh P, Feng G, et al. Efficacy and safety of topical brepocitinib cream for mild-to-moderate chronic plaque psoriasis: a phase IIb randomized double-blind vehicle-controlled parallel-group study. Br J Dermatol. 2023;189(1):33-41.
22. Worm M, Bauer A, Elsner P, Mahler V, Molin S, Nielsen TSS. Efficacy and safety of topical delgocitinib in patients with chronic hand eczema: data from a randomized, double-blind, vehicle-controlled phase IIa study. Br J Dermatol. 2020;182(5):1103-10.
23. Levy LL, Urban J, King BA. Treatment of recalcitrant atopic dermatitis with the oral Janus kinase inhibitor tofacitinib citrate. J Am Acad Dermatol. 2015;73(3):395-9.
24. Berbert Ferreira S, Berbert Ferreira R, Scheinberg MA. Atopic dermatitis: Tofacitinib, an option for refractory disease. Clin Case Rep. 2020;8(12):3244-7.
25. Komiya E, Tominaga M, Kamata Y, Suga Y, Takamori K. Molecular and Cellular Mechanisms of Itch in Psoriasis. Int J Mol Sci. 2020;21(21):8406.
26. Bachelez H, van de Kerkhof PC, Strohal R, Kubanov A, Valenzuela F, Lee JH, et al.; OPT Compare Investigators. Tofacitinib versus etanercept or placebo in moderate-to-severe chronic plaque psoriasis: a phase 3 randomised non-inferiority trial. Lancet. 2015;386(9993):552-61.
27. Papp KA, Bissonnette R, Gooderham M, et al. Treatment of plaque psoriasis with an ointment formulation of the Janus kinase inhibitor, tofacitinib: a phase 2b randomized clinical trial. BMC Dermatol. 2016;16:15.
28. Lauvelt A, Rich P, Sofen H, Strober B, Merola JF, Lebwohl M, et al. Deucravacitinib, a selective, allosteric tyrosine kinase 2 inhibitor, in scalp psoriasis: a subset analysis of two phase 3 randomized trials in plaque psoriasis. J Am Acad Dermatol. 2023:S0190-9622(23)03374-1.
29. Boch K, Langan EA, Kridin K, Zillikens D, Ludwig RJ, Bieber K. Lichen Planus. Front Med (Lausanne). 2021;8:737813.
30. Welz-Kubiak K, Reich A. Mediators of pruritus in lichen planus. Autoimmune Dis. 2013;2013:941431.
31. Bán A, Marincsák R, Bíró T, Perkecz A, Gömöri E, Sándor K, et al. Upregulation of transient receptor potential vanilloid type-1 receptor expression in oral lichen planus. Neuroimmunomodulation. 2010;17(2):103-8.
32. Abduelmula A, Bagit A, Mufti A, Yeung KCY, Yeung J. The Use of Janus Kinase Inhibitors for Lichen Planus: An Evidence-Based Review. J Cutan Med Surg. 2023;27(3):271-6.
33. Labib A, Ju T, Vander Does A, Yosipovitch G. Immunotargets and Therapy for Prurigo Nodularis. Immunotargets Ther. 2022;11:11-21.
34. Deng J, Parthasarathy V, Marani M, Bordeaux Z, Lee K, Trinh C, et al. Extracellular matrix and dermal nerve growth factor dysregulation in prurigo nodularis compared to atopic dermatitis. Front Med (Lausanne). 2022;9:1022889.
35. Ständer S, Moormann C, Schumacher M, Buddenkotte J, Artuc M, Shpacovitch V, et al. Expression of vanilloid receptor subtype 1 in cutaneous sensory nerve fibers, mast cells, and epithelial cells of appendage structures. Exp Dermatol. 2004;13(3):129-39.
36. Kwatra S, Bordeaux Z, Pritchard T, et al. Efficacy, safety, and mechanism of action of abrocitinib in the treatment of prurigo nodularis and chronic pruritus of unknown origin. Presented at: European Academy of Dermatology and Venereology Congress 2023; October 11-14, 2023. Berlin, Germany.
37. Sardana K, Sharath S, Khurana A. Use of tofacitinib in recalcitrant cases of chronic pruritus of unknown origin. Arch Dermatol Res. 2023;315(10):2955-7.

CHAPTER 10

Off-label Uses of Janus Kinase Inhibitors

Kabir Sardana

"God, grant me the serenity to accept the things I cannot change, the courage to change the things I can, and the wisdom to know the difference."
—**Serenity Prayer**

Overview

- Introduction
- Eczema
- Hidradenitis Suppurativa
- Lichen Planus
- Macrophage-activated Disorders
- Progressive Systemic Sclerosis
- Systemic Lupus Erythematosus
- Steroid-induced Rosacea
- Vasculitis and Vasculopathy

■ INTRODUCTION

Most inflammatory and autoimmune disorders have a firm immunological basis and cytokines play an important role in the mediation of these disorders. As has been detailed previously (refer to Chapters 1 and 2), many cell-to-cell interactions are mediated by cytokines. There are two families of cytokines and most of them mediate their action via Janus kinase-signal transducer and activator of transcription (JAK-STAT) receptors (Fig. 1). The naïve CD4 cell differentiates into varied subtypes and T helper 1 (Th1), Th2, Th17 cells, and JAK receptors play a role in their cytokine-mediated response. Th17 cells indirectly are affected by the JAK pathway. Hence, most disorders where cytokines have a primary or predominant role would respond to JAK inhibitor (JAKib). Notably, there are well-defined JAK pairs that mediate action of varied cytokine families, which accounts for their rapid and somewhat multicytokine action. Highly selective JAKs seem to be better and safer but except for tyrosine kinase 2 (TYK2) inhibitors most selective JAKs tend to inhibit multiple cytokines. Also the selectivity is an in vitro construct and at in vivo doses the selectivity may not prevail.

Here it is pertinent to note that while almost all inflammatory skin disorders have cytokines as a mediator, not all are amenable to JAKib. Disorders where the predominant pathway is via the CD4/CD8/cytokine axis would respond to these agents. One notable aspect that I have noted in the last 4 years of using these drugs that they do not have a long term effect, thus these drugs do not necessarily lead to long-term remissions.

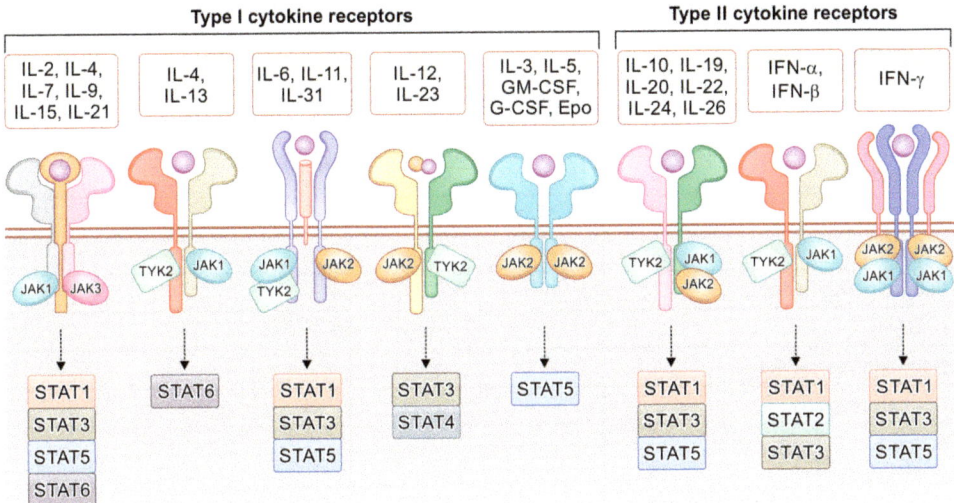

(IFN: interferon; IL: interleukin; GM-CSF: granulocyte-macrophage colony-stimulating factor; JAK: Janus kinase; STAT: signal transducer and activator of transcription; TYK2: tyrosine kinase 2)

FIG. 1: Overview of the cytokine JAK interaction.

Nevertheless they are markedly more safe and effective than oral steroids and varied oral immunosuppressive agents that dermatologists are used to prescribing, including azathioprine, cyclophosphamide, and cyclosporine.

We are detailing first a list of disorders where JAKib are useful and to make it relevant to the practicing clinicians this list is relevant to tofacitinib, which is the most cost effective JAKib in India (**Table 1**). We will be discussing a few disorders in this Chapter.

■ ECZEMA

While atopic dermatitis (AD) has been dealt with elsewhere (refer to Chapter 5), we will focus on disorders not covered in the previous chapters.

Chronic Hand Eczema

Hand eczema (HE) has a lifetime prevalence of up to 20% and a 1-year prevalence of approximately 10% in adults. There are varied risk factors associated with HE that include female sex, prior/current AD, and occupations involving exposure to irritants and/or allergens, in particular wet-work occupations. While varied morphological types have been described, which often overlap, a more useful method of classifying them is in terms of the immunology of the condition.

Thus, **allergic contact dermatitis (ACD) type** can have an immune signature that can be either Th1/Th17 in metal-induced ACD to Th2/Th22 in fragrance and rubber-induced ACD. In **ICD** Th1/Th17 is the likely cause while in the atopic variant Th2 and Th22 overexpression is seen. A recent study revealed that in chronic hand eczema (CHE) immaterial of the atopic or nonatopic nature of CHE, a predominant systemic Th2/Th1 profile was observed. As the cytokines involved mediate their effect via JAK receptors, CHE could be treated by JAKibs.[16] Notably, there is data on delgocitinib, baricitinib, upadacitinib, and recently on gusacitinib. As tofacitinib is a pan JAK, it is logical to assume that

TABLE 1	Overview of the varied indications of JAKibs and the level of evidence. As the most cost-effective option is tofacitinib, this data is derived largely from published data on this drug.	
Dermatoses	**Good quality evidence***	**Emerging role^**
Alopecia areata	✓	
Amyloidosis		✓[1]
ABCD		✓[2]
Behçet	✓[3]	
Bullous pemphigoid		✓
CAD		✓
Dermatitis herpetiformis		✓
Dermatomyositis[4]	✓	
Eczema: • Atopic dermatitis • Discoid eczema • Chronic hand eczema	✓	 ✓ ✓
Erythema multiforme	✓[5]	
Epidermolysis bullosa pruriginosa		✓
Granuloma annulare	✓[6]	
Hidradenitis suppurativa		✓[7]
Hypereosinophilic syndrome		✓
Itch		✓[8]
Keloid		✓[9]
Leukocytoclastic vasculitis		✓
Lupus erythematosus	✓[10]	
LMDF		✓
Lichen planus		✓
Linear IgA BD		✓
LSCEA		✓
Morphea		✓
Morbihan disease		✓
Netherton syndrome		✓
NLD	✓	
Pyoderma gangrenosum	✓	
PLCA		✓[11]
PMLE		✓[12]
Prurigo nodularis	✓	
PPK		✓
PRP		✓
Psoriasis	✓[13]	

Continued

Continued

Dermatoses	Good quality evidence*	Emerging role^
PSS	✓	
Rosacea		✓[14]
Sarcoidosis	✓	
Scabies nodular		✓
Steroid-induced rosacea		✓[15]
Urticaria		✓
Vitiligo		✓
Vasculitis		✓
Vasculopathy		✓

* Long-term data and cytokine based translational studies.
^ Case reports and case series

(BD: bullous dermatosis; CAD: coronary artery disease; IgA: immunoglobulin A; JAKibs: Janus kinase inhibitors; NLD: necrobiosis lipoidica; LMDF: lupus miliaris disseminatus faciei; LSCEA: lichen sclerous et atrophicus; PLCA: primary localized cutaneous amyloidosis; PMLE: polymorphic light eruption; PRP: platelet-rich plasma; PPK: plantar keratoderma; PSS: progressive systemic sclerosis)

TABLE 2	JAKibs trialed in chronic hand eczema.
Topical	**Mode of action**
• Delgocitinib	• Pan-JAK (JAK1, 2, 3, and TYK2)
• Ruxolitinib	• Selective JAK1 and 2
• Tofacitinib	• JAK1, 3 > 2
Systemic	**Mode of action**
• Gusacitinib	• JAK/SYK (JAK1/JAK2/JAK3 + TYK2 and SYK)
• Upadacitinib	• Selective JAK1
• Baricitinib	• JAK1/2
• Abrocitinib	• JAK1

(CHE: chronic hand eczema; JAKib: Janus kinase inhibitor; SYK: spleen tyrosine kinase; TYK2: tyrosine kinase 2)

this drug also be useful in CHE. A summary of the various JAKib trialed in CHE is listed in **Table 2**.

Notably, general measures that apply to cases of CHE including barrier measures and topical glucocorticoids (GCs) are still essential and can help sustain the effect of JAKibs. As of today this class of drugs are reserved for severe CHE, but with rising evidence that shows that Th1 and Th2 pathways play a prominent role in most forms of CHE, this class of drugs may replace existing systemic agents.

■ HIDRADENITIS SUPPURATIVA[7]

Hidradenitis suppurativa (HS) is a disorder where the ideal medical therapy is difficult to determine even though most clinicians use oral antibiotics, acitretin, metformin, and biologicals while possibly the ideal modality might be surgical intervention as most patients come to dermatologists late in an advanced stage of the disease. Nevertheless cytokines-based therapy has been administered with both tumor necrosis factor alpha (TNF-α) and interleukin 17 (IL-17) being the targeted cytokines.

TABLE 3	Clinical trials of JAKib in HS.			
JAKibs	Target	Administration	Phase	Study number/sponsor
Tofacitinib	JAK1, JAK3	Oral	Phase 2	NCT04246372 University of Colorado, Denver
Upadacitinib	JAK1	Oral	Phase 3	NCT05889182 AbbVie
Deucravacitinib	TYK2	Oral	Phase 2	NCT05997277 Beth Israel Deaconess Medical Center

(HS: hidradenitis suppurativa; JAKib: Janus kinase inhibitor; TYK2: tyrosine kinase 2)

Among the JAKibs to date, there is only one published clinical trial in the literature, a real-life study with 15 patients up to week 24 in which upadacitinib was used and a case series where tofacitinib was successfully used. Conversely, there are several ongoing clinical trials (**Table 3**). Unless we perform trials based on the stage and severity of HS, JAKib as a class may be at best an adjunctive drug. In this authors experience, tofacitinib is not effective in HS.

LICHEN PLANUS

Lichen Planus Immunopathogenesis

After antigenic stimulation, there is a differentiation of the effector T lymphocytes that are predominantly composed of Th1 and Th17 lymphocytes, which are stimulated by interferon gamma (IFN-γ) and IL-17. Apart from the cytokines released by these cells, CD8+ lymphocytes (Tc1 and Tc17) mediate epidermal injury by the "Fas-Fas ligand" (FasL) and "TNF-α-TNF-α receptors" interaction and also by release of cytotoxic molecules such as perforin, granzyme B, and granulysin, which in turn lead to keratinocyte apoptosis with consequent epidermal and dermal changes.

The main cell lines are the CD4+ and CD8+ T lymphocytes and their related cytokines. The increased number of CD4+ T lymphocytes creates a band-like infiltrate in the subepidermal area and it has been suggested that the increased CD4+ T lymphocyte infiltration is associated with a better and sustained response to therapy. Th1 lymphocytes secrete **IFN-γ, IL-2, and TNF-α** and activate macrophages and CD8+ T lymphocytes. Th2, Th9, and Th17 lymphocytes release **IL-26, IL-22, and IL-17** and serve as drivers of the chronic tissue inflammatory response. Notably, **IFN-γ, IL-2, IL-26, and IL-22** mediate their action via JAK receptors.

The use of JAKib thus is based on firm evidence as these drugs block the salient cytokines.[17] There are multiple reports of successful use of baricitinib and tofacitinib in erosive, palmoplantar,[18] nail,[19] and hypertrophic LP.[20] Ideally though the cytokine profile predicts the efficacy of JAKibs and can explain the lack of response in certain cases of LP. In our experience most cases of LP respond to tofacitinib, especially oral LP while it should be reserved for difficult variants like lichen planus hypertrophicus (LPH) (**Figs. 2A to D**).

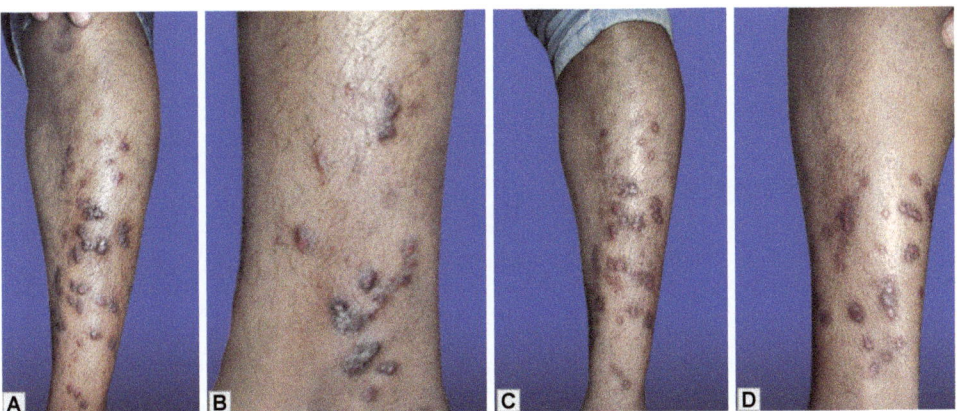

(LPH: lichen planus hypertrophicus; OMP: oral minipulse; TCS: topical corticosteroid)

FIGS. 2A TO D: (A and B) A case of LPH who had failed OMP, methotrexate, and dapsone. In addition to TCS, tofacitinib was initiated in a dose of 5 mg BD. (C and D) After 6 weeks of therapy, there is marked improvement.

■ MACROPHAGE-ACTIVATED DISORDERS

Granuloma Annulare, Necrobiosis Lipoidica, and Sarcoidosis

Background[21]

CD4+ helper T cells are the predominant lymphocyte population associated with both infectious and noninfectious granulomatous inflammation and secrete high levels of IFN-γ, other cytokines such as IL-2 and IL-17, and monocyte-recruiting chemokines. IFN-γ along with CD40 ligand (CD40L) appears to play a prominent functional role in inflammatory polarization of macrophages and granuloma formation in vivo in mouse models and macrophages have been shown to produce IL-6, IL-12, IL-18, IL-23, TNF-α, and T-cell chemokines. These mutually-reinforcing cytokine programs likely create a self-sustaining loop perpetuating granulomatous inflammation in the presence of pathogenic antigens. Medications that disrupt these cytokine-based communication networks between T cells and macrophages might be an effective treatment approach in these disorders.

Macrophages play a key role in many functions including immunity and tissue homeostasis/repair. While macrophages are likely important in the pathogenesis of many autoimmune diseases, in a subset of these disorders, macrophage activation and accumulation in tissue is a central pathogenic feature. These disorders include granuloma annulare (GA) and necrobiosis lipoidica (NL) that affect the skin, Crohn's disease (CD) that affects the gastrointestinal tract, and sarcoidosis that can affect nearly any organ system and is often present in multiple organ systems simultaneously (most commonly the lungs, lymph nodes, and/or skin). Hemophagocytic lymphohistiocytosis (HLH) is a syndrome characterized by systemic macrophage activation.

Granuloma Annulare

There has been a study where tissue cytokine expression was performed, which revealed that GA lesions expressed *IFN-γ*, which was secreted by CD4+ T cells and was associated with inflammatory polarization of macrophages and fibroblasts. In particular, macrophages upregulate oncostatin M, an IL-6 family cytokine, which appears to act on fibroblasts to alter

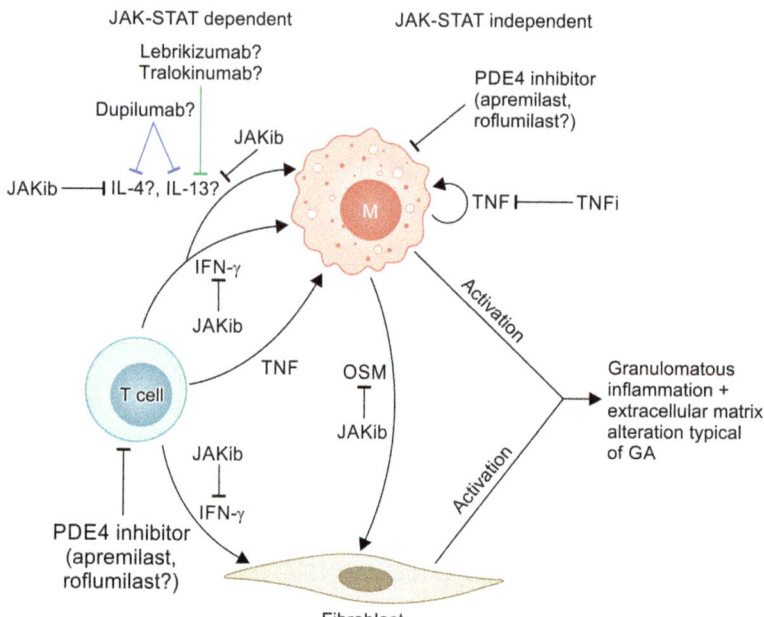

(GA: granuloma annulare; IFN: interferon; JAKib: Janus kinase inhibitor; OSM: oncostatin M; PDE4: phosphodiesterase-4; STAT: signal transducer and activator of transcription; TNFi: tumor necrosis factor inhibitor)

FIG. 3: Cytokines that mediate pathogenesis of GA and the role of varied oral agents in its treatment.

extracellular matrix production, a hallmark of GA. *IL-15 and IL-21* production appeared to feedback on CD4+ T cells to sustain inflammation (**Fig. 3**).

Notably, the implicated cytokines mediate their action via JAK1/2 (IFN-γ) and via JAK1/3 (IL-15/IL-21), which makes it an ideal disorder where JAKib can be effective. Proof-of-concept studies by Wang A et al. have shown that the use of **oral tofacitinib** is useful and mirrors the cytokine suppression. A higher dose of tofacitinib up to 20 mg may be needed in certain cases. Other JAKib have also been tried including upadacitinib and baricitinib. There are as yet no intraclass studies to suggest the ideal JAKib.

Sarcoidosis

The varied cytokines implicated in sarcoidosis including type I IFNs (IFN-α/β), IFN-γ, IL-6, IL-12, IL-23, and granulocyte-macrophage colony-stimulating factor (GM-CSF), which signal through the JAK-STAT pathway. Depending on the specificity of the JAKib employed, some or many of these cytokines could be simultaneously inhibited. Other cytokines such as IL-17 and TNF do not signal directly through the JAK pathway but as TNF-α is secreted by CD4 Th1 cells, which are in turn is stimulated by IL-12 and INF-γ, which mediate their action via the JAK-STAT pathway; this seems to be a target for JAKib.

There is data that has shown clinical efficacy for both cutaneous and pulmonary sarcoidosis with JAKibs, including **tofacitinib** ($n = 23$), **ruxolitinib** ($n = 3$), and **baricitinib** ($n = 1$) with majority of patients achieving complete or near-complete resolution of their cutaneous disease.

Prurigo Nodularis

Background and Immunopathogenesis

This disorder is believed to be consequent to a combination of both immunological and neurological activation both at a central and peripheral level. Skin lesions in prurigo nodularis (PN) demonstrate increases in cutaneous nerve fiber density, immune cell infiltration, and cytokine expression in addition to epidermal hyperplasia and hyperkeratosis (Fig. 4).

In the skin, keratinocytes communicate with sensory nerve endings, especially pruriceptors, via synaptic-like contacts. Itch perception and the appearance of prurigo lesions are related to these interactions, with a role of mast cells, eosinophils, dendritic cells (DCs), or T lymphocytes. Studies have revealed that three pruriceptive nerve-ending populations can be identified in mice: MrgprD+ neurons; neurons expressing MrgprA3, MrgprC11, histamine receptors, and the IL-33 receptor; and nerve endings expressing serotonin receptors and the IL-31 receptor. In humans, MrgpRX2 is highly expressed in lesions. IL-4 and IL-13 receptors are detected in all three neurons. In mice, scratching behaviors have been shown to vary according to the activation of these different subtypes.

In prurigo lesions, **Th2** cytokines, especially **IL-31**,[22] seem to be the key cytokine and it bridges the gap between immune cells, the nervous system, and the skin. IL-31 is a cytokine secreted predominantly by CD4+ T cells specifically the Th2 cells. The receptor for IL-31 is composed of two subunits, IL-31 receptor A (IL-31RA) and oncostatin M receptor β (OSMRβ), and signals through a downstream JAK-STAT3 pathway via the JAK1/2/TYK2 pathway. IL-31 receptor A is expressed on sensory neurons, keratinocytes, and myeloid cells, and IL-31RA/ORMRβ signaling is thought to potentiate the itch, epidermal hyperplasia, and inflammation in PN (Fig. 4).[23] Specifically, IL-31RA is expressed on a subset of small C-fiber neurons that innervate the skin from the dorsal root ganglion (DRG). IL-31 signaling to DRG neurons leads to neuronal activation, axonal outgrowth, and

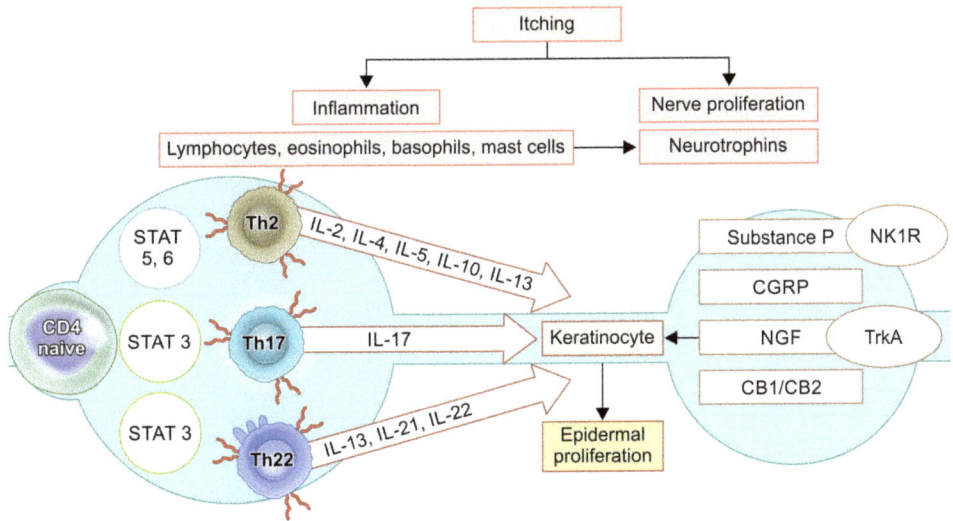

(IL: interleukin; NK1R: neurokinin-1 receptor; STAT: signal transducer and activator of transcription; Th: T helper)

FIG. 4: An overview of the pathogenesis of prurigo nodularis.

scratching. Another cytokine implicated is **IL-4,** which cannot induce itch, but is thought to enhance neuronal responsiveness to pruritogens such as histamine and IL-31 to promote chronic itch.

A systemic and cutaneous **Th22 and Th17** immune polarization of PN has also been characterized in certain studies.

Therapies

The therapies can be divided into two categories:
1. **Neuromodulating therapies** naloxone, naltrexone, and nalbuphine, neurokinin-1 (NK1) receptor (NK1R) antagonists like aprepitant and serlopitant, antidepressants like paroxetine, fluvoxamine and duloxetine, and gabapentinoids.
2. **Immunomodulating therapies** biologics like dupilumab, nemolizumab, and oral JAKibs

Of these the salient drugs that work on the major immune mediators are listed in the **Table 4.**

Notably while dupilumab has been Food and Drug Administration (FDA) approved, its action is identical to that of tofacitinib and like in AD, tofacitinib has been found to be as effective as dupilumab,[24] which is in any case prohibitively costly in India. A recent study has found that JAKib (baricitinib and upadacitinib 15 mg daily) achieved identical results as compared to dupilumab.[24]

The action of JAKib unlike biologicals works across cytokine families and as has been seen in AD trials these drugs are comparable in efficacy to biologicals. Our own experience has been largely with tofacitinib,[20,21] which has helped in managing severe case of PN even without the use of antihistamines, which suggest that it could eventually replace the present therapies in PN (**Figs. 5A and B**).

TABLE 4	Overview of novel therapeutic agents in PN.	
Th2 cytokines and receptors		
IL-4R/IL-13R	Dupilumab	Dupilumab 300 mg (loading dose 600 mg) SC Q2W for 24 weeks
IL-31RA	Nemolizumab	Nemolizumab 0.5 mg/kg SC at baseline, week 4 and week 8
OSMRβ	Vixarelimab (KPL-716)	Vixarelimab 360 mg SC weekly (loading dose 720 mg SC)
JAK and tyrosine kinase KIT receptors		
JAK1/3	Tofacitinib	• Dose 5–15 mg[25-27] • Marked reduction in itching and clinical resolution in most cases by 3–4 weeks
JAK1	Abrocitinib	Abrocitinib 200 mg orally daily
JAK1	Povorcitinib	Recruiting
Tyrosine kinase KIT receptor	Barzolvolimab	Single dose IV

(IL: interleukin; IL-31RA: IL-31 receptor A; JAK: Janus kinase; OSMRβ: oncostatin M receptor β; PN: prurigo nodularis; SC: subcutaneous)

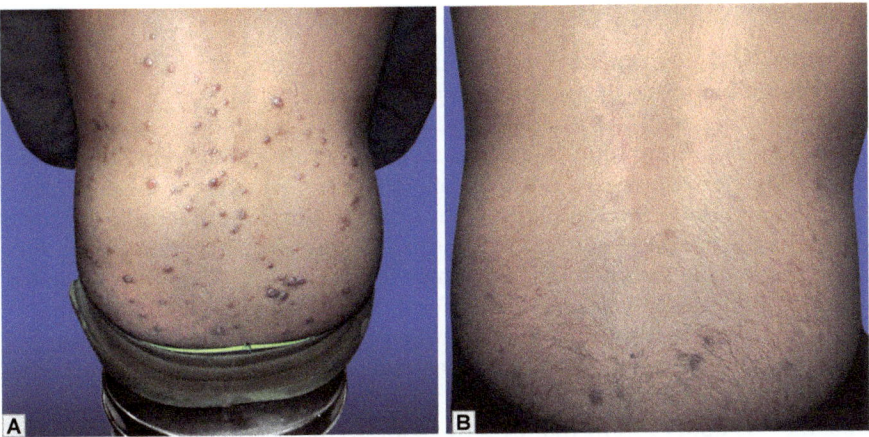

FIGS. 5A AND B: A generalized case of prurigo nodularis (PN) in an adolescent and response after 12 weeks of tofacitinib 5 mg BD. (Indian J Dermatol Venereol Leprol. 2023:1-3.)

■ PROGRESSIVE SYSTEMIC SCLEROSIS

While there are multiple pathways for the causation of progressive systemic sclerosis (PSS), we will focus on the immunological pathway.[28] B cells from systemic sclerosis (SSc) patients not only produce autoantibodies, but can also infiltrate tissues and show increased activation markers such as CD19, CD21, costimulatory molecules, and B-cell activating factor (BAFF). There is evidence in murine models that overexpression of CD19 induces the production of cutaneous fibrosis and that the absence of B cells is associated with decreased fibrosis.

The T lymphocytes from SSc patients show an increased expression of activation markers. Th2 cells, producing **IL-4 and IL-13**, and Th17, producing IL-17, are increased in both skin and peripheral blood of patients with SSc, particularly in patients with the diffuse form of the disease. Varied immune system cells, such as macrophages and DCs, can also infiltrate skin of SSc patients, producing proinflammatory and profibrotic cytokines and chemokines, which in turn are responsible for the process of endothelial-mesenchymal transition (EMT). Thus these cells transform into myofibroblasts.

Although the factors that promote the persistent activation of cells of the immune system are unknown, recent studies have highlighted the possible role of toll-like receptors (TLRs) in the activation of DCs, which could in turn secrete proinflammatory cytokines and present antigens to the T cells. Overexpression of TLR4 and TLR2 has been found in skin and fibroblasts of patients with SSc. Activation of DCs through TLRs generally leads to the production of several proinflammatory cytokines, particularly **type I IFN**, which have been found overexpressed in the sera of patients with SSc and 50% of SSc patients may show this so-called "interferon signature" in the peripheral blood. These are seen in the early phase, before overt skin fibrosis.

Interleukin 33 an alarmin of the IL-1 family related to inflammation and fibrosis has been recently implicated in the pathogenesis of SSc. Following the production of IL-33 and IL-25 by innate lymphoid cells, there is an overproduction of IL-4 and IL-13 that increases collagen deposition by fibroblasts and induces the differentiation of macrophages toward a profibrotic phenotype.

Role of Janus Kinase Pathway

The activation of IL-12 cytokine family exerts a mainly profibrotic effect. **IL-4, IL-5, and IL-13** cytokines belong to the γ chain receptor subfamily and exert a profibrotic effect that may be blocked via **JAK1 and JAK3** inhibitors, resulting in the reduced polarization of Th cells toward a profibrotic Th2 response. Similarly, the IL-12 cytokines, **IL-23 and IL-27**, are characterized by a significant profibrotic effect. The role of the last member of the IL-12 family, IL-35, is characterized by dual profibrotic and antifibrotic activity. Therefore, the net effect depends on which signaling pathway is predominantly blocked. JAKis can block signaling via the IFN receptor that translates to a reduction in the IFN signature (and a potential therapeutic effect). **IL-10** cytokine family members exert both antifibrotic (IL-10) as well as strong profibrotic effects (IL-31). In line with this, the inhibition of the IL-10 family's signaling may exaggerate the profibrotic effect when the IL-10 signaling is blocked.

While there is data to show that JAKi (tofacitinib) may help in reducing the sclerosis and the early radiological abnormalities in SSc-interstitial lung disease (ILD) patients larger studies are needed, particularly to understand at what stage of the disease would these drugs effectively halt or reverse the disease process. A meta-analysis[29] that studied 59 cases found that the duration of therapy needed was 12 (6–12) months. The JAKibs (tofacitinib in 47 patients and baricitinib in 12 patients) were prescribed as first-line therapy in 35 patients (59%). A significant cutaneous response [decrease in the mRSS (modified Rodnan skin score) of >5 points and ≥25% from baseline) was reported in 52 patients (88%). Among patients with ILD ($n = 31$), majority had no disease progression. Cutaneous response was more frequently observed in treatment naïve SSc patients. While more data is awaited JAKib seems to be an ideal drug that target both the immunological pathway and consequent fibrosis.

■ SYSTEMIC LUPUS ERYTHEMATOSUS

Systemic lupus erythematosus (SLE) is a multisystem autoimmune disease that is more common in women (particularly those of reproductive age) than in men, and that can affect the skin, joints, heart, kidneys, serosa, nerves, and blood vessels, presenting with a variety of clinical symptoms. It is pathologically characterized by activation of **autoreactive T cells** and production of autoantibodies by **B cells**.

Glucocorticoids and conventional immunosuppressants are widely used treatments, but their targets are nonspecific, and effective targeted therapies are needed. Many SLE disease-susceptibility genes identified by genome-wide association study (GWAS) are highly expressed in adaptive immune cells, including B cells, and B-cell activation processes, and overproduction of autoantibodies are notable pathological features of SLE. The B cells further differentiate into autoantibody-producing cells in response to IL-21 and other cytokines. In addition, B cells produce various cytokines, such as IL-6. Thus, the therapy of SLE revolves around B cell inhibition.

Genome-wide association studies have resulted in identification of the genes encoding IL-1 receptor-associated kinase 1, IFN regulatory factor 5, TLR-7, TYK2, and STAT4 as disease-susceptibility genes for SLE. Thus, there is also an overproduction of IFNs and the concomitant overexpression of IFN-induced genes (known as the "interferon signature"), which is highly expressed on DCs. TLRs are highly expressed in DCs in patients with SLE, and their contribution to aberrant cell death, including neutrophil death through formation of neutrophil extracellular traps (NETs), induces the production of cytokines and chemokines, which has an important role in triggering subsequent loss of immune tolerance. The **cytokines**, which are produced by the innate immune system, include soluble BAFF, type I IFNs, type II IFN, type III IFNs, and IL-12 and/or IL-23, which in turn induce the differentiation and activation of T cells, and lead to class switching and differentiation of B cells to autoantibody-producing cells in the adaptive immune system. Thus, these cytokines link the innate and adaptive immune systems and are of particular interest as targets for treatment.

The use of JAKibs in SLE is currently being assessed. Cytokines that bridge the innate and adaptive immune systems, such as **type I IFNs, IL-12, and IL-23**, as well as those that activate T cell–B cell interaction, such as **IL-21, IL-6** and **IL-4**, are likely targets of JAKibs in SLE.[30]

Multiple trials are being conducted in LE including DLE and it is yet to be seen whether this class of drugs can be used as monotherapy or as an adjuvant to existing drugs.

■ STEROID-INDUCED ROSACEA

Steroid-induced rosacea (SIR) is a severe withdrawal reaction that occurs after long-term and excessive topical steroids application on face is discontinued, resembling rosacea that can present erubescence, angiotelectasis, and pustules. Avoidance of application of steroids to the face and the use of topical antibiotics, tetracycline antibiotics, and antihistamines have traditionally been the treatment options, which turn out to be insufficient.

While in India we use the term topical steroid damaged face (TSDF), it is an unnecessary name as SIR is a well-established terminology and the only difference is the presence of signs of steroid overuse in TSDF. A recent study found that mometasone in the form "No-Scar" preparation was the most commonly abused topical steroid. Apart from steroid-induced acne (45.2%) or flare of preexisting acne, the next common feature was erythema and telangiectasia (21.2%), hypertrichosis (6.6%), rosacea (2.2%), and atrophy (1.5%).[31] The paradox of GCs causing increase inflammation in rosacea and perioral dermatitis has been explained by the fact that they increase the expression of proinflammatory cytokine CCL20, via recruiting Th17 and this is elevated in papulopustular rosacea.[32] A further theory suggests that steroids augment TLR2 expression in human keratinocytes, which enhances kallikrein-related peptidase 5 production and activity, turning cathelicidin into the activated form LL-37. LL-37 contributes to the telangiectasia and angiogenesis in epidermis and aggravates inflammatory response with emergence of proinflammatory cytokines (e.g., TNF-α, IL-6, and IL-8). Notably, all these cytokines mediate their action via the JAK pathway.

There are now two case series with successful use of JAKib in SIR. In the first case tofacitinib was used in a dose of 5 mg BD, which showed a marked response in 2 weeks and was further tapered down over 4 weeks with marked resolution of lesions.[15] The second series used abrocitinib with similar results.[33]

■ VASCULITIS AND VASCULOPATHY

Etiopathogenesis

Cell-mediated, immune complex-mediated, and antineutrophil cytoplasmic antibody (ANCA)-associated mechanisms are involved depending on the vasculitis. Examples of **cell-mediated vasculitis** include giant cell arteritis (GCA), Takayasu arteritis, and primary central nervous system (CNS) vasculitis. Examples of **immune complex**-mediated vasculitis include polyarteritis nodosa (PAN), Henoch–Schönlein purpura, cryoglobulinemic vasculitis, and cutaneous leukocytoclastic angiitis. The ANCA-associated vasculitides, which may involve **both** cellular and humoral mechanisms, include granulomatosis with polyangiitis (GPA; Wegener granulomatosis), microscopic polyangiitis (MPA), and eosinophilic GPA (EGPA; Churg–Strauss syndrome). The immune mechanisms of the other types of vasculitis are less certain.

As there is a predominant role of lymphocytes and cytokines, JAK receptors play a dominant role. A recent paper[34] examined the JAK expression in cutaneous vasculitis and found an increased expression of JAK1 and JAK2 in the development of cutaneous symptoms of IgA vasculitis (IgAV) and cutaneous leukocytoclastic vasculitis (CLV). Also serum levels of IFN-γ, IL-6, and IL-23 are elevated in patients with IgAV. As noted in **Figure 1**, IFN-γ signals through JAK1-JAK2, IL-6 through JAK1-JAK2-TYK2, and IL-23 through JAK2-TYK2, whereas IL-4 and IL-13 signal through JAK1-JAK3 or JAK1-TYK2. Thus, this shows that JAK inhibition would be effective in vasculitis.

Treatment

Small-vessel vasculitis confined to the skin usually needs less aggressive treatment than systemic vasculitis involving large- and/or medium-sized arteries. Large-vessel vasculitis is treated initially with GCs. There is a need for steroid-sparing agents and apart from the conventional ISA and biologic therapy (e.g., tocilizumab for GCA) there is increasing evidence for the use of baricitinib/tofacitinib, which has shown great effectiveness enabling rapid tapering of GCs and reduction of steroid side effects.[35] Similar results have been noted in Takayasu arteritis.[36]

In case of ANCA the combination of cyclophosphamide and prednisone is often regarded as the first choice for induction therapy of generalized and severe types of medium and ANCA-associated vasculitis. New targeted biologic agents may replace cyclophosphamide as induction therapy for some forms of vasculitis (e.g., rituximab for GPA and MPA, mepolizumab for EGPA). Maintenance therapies are less well defined but typically involve the use of azathioprine, methotrexate, or mycophenolate mofetil. Again there are reports of the use of tofacitinib in ANCA-associated vasculitis.[37]

Thus, while small vessel vasculitis[38] is amenable to JAKibs, they can be used as adjuncts to existing therapies in case of failures to the primary therapy.

■ CONCLUSION

A host of disorders are amenable to JAKib (**Table 1**). The spectrum of potential usage is vast and extends beyond the approved uses of AA, AD, and psoriatic arthritis (PsoA). Notably in almost all the approved indications tofacitinib is effective being a pan JAKib. The premise of selectivity is based on in vitro data and may not necessarily be applicable at clinical doses. Nevertheless, for now as clinicians we can reserve the drug in disorders where existing drugs fail, but there is little justification in adhering to long-term steroids or oral minipulse (OMP), the latter is anyways not based on sound pharmacological principles. Pulse is a dose of >100 mg prednisolone and long-acting steroids used in a low-dose fashion can cause side-effects. The OMP was based more on dose availability and cost than any pharmacological logic. If such a regimen is to be given, it is better to use a short-acting or intermediate-acting steroid, like m-prednisolone in an alternate day regimen. In any case JAKibs are immensely more specific than steroids and can replace them in most chronic inflammatory disorders.

There is an urgent need for tissue cytokine and JAK-based data to arrive at the ideal JAKib drug and such translational data can be useful for clinicians. Such data (**Fig. 1**) translates into uses which will achieve a high degree of credibility (**Table 1**) and success and there is a need for more data from India on this important aspect. Tofacitinib is a remarkably well-tolerated drug and would eventually replace ISA and possibly steroids in many autoimmune skin disorders.

■ REFERENCES

1. Chen J, Yang B. Tofacitinib for the treatment of primary cutaneous amyloidosis: A case report. Dermatol Ther. 2022;35(4):e15312.
2. Muddebihal A, Sardana K, Sinha S, Kumar D. Tofacitinib in refractory Parthenium-induced airborne allergic contact dermatitis. Contact Dermatitis. 2023;88(2):150-2.
3. Liu J, Hou Y, Sun L, Li C, Li L, Zhao Y, et al. A pilot study of tofacitinib for refractory Behçet's syndrome. Ann Rheum Dis. 2020;79(11):1517-20.
4. Zhang J, Sun L, Shi X, Li S, Liu C, Li X, et al. Janus kinase inhibitor, tofacitinib, in refractory juvenile dermatomyositis: a retrospective multi-central study in China. Arthritis Res Ther. 2023;25(1):204.
5. Murphy MJ, Gruenstein D, Wang A, Peterson D, Levitt J, King B, et al. Treatment of Persistent Erythema Multiforme With Janus Kinase Inhibition and the Role of Interferon Gamma and Interleukin 15 in Its Pathogenesis. JAMA Dermatol. 2021;157(12):1477-82.
6. Wang A, Rahman NT, McGeary MK, Murphy M, McHenry A, Peterson D, et al. Treatment of granuloma annulare and suppression of proinflammatory cytokine activity with tofacitinib. J Allergy Clin Immunol. 2021;147(5):1795-809.
7. Heidari A, Ghane Y, Heidari N, Sadeghi S, Goodarzi A. A systematic review of Janus kinase inhibitors and spleen tyrosine kinase inhibitors for Hidradenitis suppurativa treatment. Int Immunopharmacol. 2023;127:111435.
8. Sardana K, Sharath S, Khurana A. Use of tofacitinib in recalcitrant cases of chronic pruritus of unknown origin. Arch Dermatol Res. 2023;315(10):2955-7.
9. Chen JY, Feng QL, Pan HH, Zhu DH, He RL, Deng CC, et al. An Open-Label, Uncontrolled, Single-Arm Clinical Trial of Tofacitinib, an Oral JAK1 and JAK3 Kinase Inhibitor, in Chinese Patients with Keloid. Dermatology. 2023;239(5):818-27.
10. Nikolopoulos D, Parodis I. Janus kinase inhibitors in systemic lupus erythematosus: implications for tyrosine kinase 2 inhibition. Front Med (Lausanne). 2023;10:1217147.
11. Chen J, Yang B. Tofacitinib for the treatment of primary cutaneous amyloidosis: A case report. Dermatol Ther. 2022;35(4):e15312.
12. Sardana K, Mathachan SR, Khurana A. Tofacitinib: A Treatment Option for Recalcitrant Polymorphic Light Eruption and Its Mechanistic Rationale. Dermatitis. 2024. [Online ahead of print]
13. Megna M, Potestio L, Ruggiero A, Cacciapuoti S, Maione F, Tasso M, et al. JAK Inhibitors in Psoriatic Disease. Clin Cosmet Investig Dermatol. 2023;16:3129-45.
14. Sun YH, Man XY, Xuan XY, Huang CZ, Shen Y, Lao LM. Tofacitinib for the treatment of erythematotelangiectatic and papulopustular rosacea: A retrospective case series. Dermatol Ther. 2022;35(11):e15848.
15. Li T, Wang H, Wang C, Hao P. Tofacitinib for the Treatment of Steroid-Induced Rosacea. Clin Cosmet Investig Dermatol. 2022;15:2519-21.
16. Ho JS, Molin S. A review of existing and new treatments for the management of hand eczema. J Cutan Med Surg. 2023;27(5):493-503.
17. Schinner J, Cunha T, Mayer JU, Hörster S, Kind P, Didona D, et al. Skin-infiltrating T cells display distinct inflammatory signatures in lichen planus, bullous pemphigoid and pemphigus vulgaris. Front Immunol. 2023;14:1203776.
18. Bazargan AS, Jafarzadeh A, Nobari NN. Successful treatment of resistant plantar ulcerative lichen planus with tofacitinib: A case report and comprehensive review of the literature. Clin Case Rep. 2023;11(10):e8066.
19. Huang J, Shi W. Successful treatment of nail lichen planus with tofacitinib: a case report and review of the literature. Front Med (Lausanne). 2023;10:1301123.
20. Abduelmula A, Bagit A, Mufti A, Yeung KCY, Yeung J. The Use of Janus Kinase Inhibitors for Lichen Planus: An Evidence-Based Review. J Cutan Med Surg. 2023;27(3):271-6.
21. Wang A, Singh K, Ibrahim W, King B, Damsky W. The Promise of JAK Inhibitors for Treatment of Sarcoidosis and Other Inflammatory Disorders with Macrophage Activation: A Review of the Literature. Yale J Biol Med. 2020;93(1):187-95.

22. Datsi A, Steinhoff M, Ahmad F, Alam M, Buddenkotte J. Interleukin-31: the "itchy" cytokine in inflammation and therapy. Allergy. 2021;76(10):2982-97.
23. Kashem SW, Fassett MS. Can Serum Biomarkers for Prurigo Nodularis Expose Pathophysiology or Just Treatment Response? JAMA Dermatol. 2023;159(9):915-7.
24. Yew YW, Yeo PM. Comparison between dupilumab and oral Janus kinase inhibitors in the treatment of prurigo nodularis with or without atopic dermatitis in a tertiary care center in Singapore. JAAD Int. 2023;13:13-4.
25. Sardana K, Rose Mathachan S, Agrawal D. Treatment of recalcitrant paediatric prurigo nodularis with tofacitinib, an exquisite example of bench-to-bedside translation of JAK-STAT expression. Indian J Dermatol Venereol Leprol. 2023:1-3.
26. Agrawal D, Sardana K, Mathachan SR, Ahuja A. A Case of Recalcitrant Prurigo Nodularis with Heightened Expression of STAT 3 and STAT 6 and its Dramatic Response to Tofacitinib. Indian Dermatol Online J. 2023;14(4):564-6.
27. Liu T, Chu Y, Wang Y, Zhong X, Yang C, Bai J, et al. Successful treatment of prurigo nodularis with tofacitinib: The experience from a single center. Int J Dermatol. 2023;62(5):e293-e295.
28. Benfaremo D, Svegliati S, Paolini C, Agarbati S, Moroncini G. Systemic Sclerosis: From Pathophysiology to Novel Therapeutic Approaches. Biomedicines. 2022;10(1):163.
29. Moriana C, Moulinet T, Jaussaud R, Decker P. JAK inhibitors and systemic sclerosis: A systematic review of the literature. Autoimmun Rev. 2022;21(10):103168.
30. Tanaka Y, Luo Y, O'Shea JJ, Nakayamada S. Janus kinase-targeting therapies in rheumatology: a mechanisms-based approach. Nat Rev Rheumatol. 2022;18(3):133-45.
31. Jain S, Mohapatra L, Mohanty P, Jena S, Behera B. Study of Clinical Profile of Patients Presenting with Topical Steroid-Induced Facial Dermatosis to a Tertiary Care Hospital. Indian Dermatol Online J. 2020;11(2):208-11.
32. Wang L, Yang M, Wang X, Cheng B, Ju Q, Eichenfield DZ, et al. Glucocorticoids promote CCL20 expression in keratinocytes. Br J Dermatol. 2021;185(6):1200-8.
33. Xu B, Xu Z, Ye S, Sun H, Zhao B, Wu N, et al. JAK1 inhibitor abrocitinib for the treatment of steroid-induced rosacea: case series. Front Med (Lausanne). 2023;10:1239869.
34. Ebata A, Ogawa-Momohara M, Fukaura R, Yamashita Y, Koizumi H, Takeichi T, et al. Increased Janus kinase activation in cutaneous vasculitis. J Am Acad Dermatol. 2023:S0190-9622(23)03109-2.
35. Eriksson P, Skoglund O, Hemgren C, Sjöwall C. Clinical experience and safety of Janus kinase inhibitors in giant cell arteritis: a retrospective case series from Sweden. Front Immunol. 2023;14:1187584.
36. Mv P, Maikap D, Padhan P. Successful Use of Tofacitinib in Refractory Takayasu Arteritis: A Case Series. Mediterr J Rheumatol. 2023;34(3):356-62.
37. Liu Y, Ji Z, Yu W, Wu S, Chen H, Ma L, et al. Tofacitinib for the treatment of antineutrophil cytoplasm antibody-associated vasculitis: a pilot study. Ann Rheum Dis. 2021;80(12):1631-3.
38. Zhu KJ, Yang PD, Xu Q. Tofacitinib Treatment of Refractory Cutaneous Leukocytoclastic Vasculitis: A Case Report. Front Immunol. 2021;12:695768.

CHAPTER 11

Adverse Effects of JAK Inhibitors

Varadraj V Pai, Amrutha Solanke

"Life does not get in the way; it is the way."
—Rebecca Li, "Translating Silence"

Overview

- Introduction
- Adverse Effects
- Systemic Side Effects of Janus Kinase Inhibitors

■ INTRODUCTION

Janus kinase (JAK) is a family of intracellular, nonreceptor tyrosine kinases that transduce cytokine-mediated signals via the JAK-signal transducer and activator of transcription (JAK-STAT) pathway. They are arranged as identical homodimers (e.g., JAK2/JAK2) or heterodimers (e.g., JAK1/JAK3) bound to the cell surface receptor (**Fig. 1**). Binding of a number of cytokines and growth factors to this cell surface receptors results in phosphorylation of receptor-associated JAKs. Phosphorylation activates the JAKs, and they, in turn, phosphorylate intracellular components of the receptors, which enables recruitment of transcription factors of the STAT family. Activated STAT proteins translocate to the nucleus and induce transcription.

Intracellular signal transduction involves combinations of four JAK isoforms [JAK1, JAK2, JAK3, and tyrosine kinase 2 (TYK2)] and seven STAT family members. The usage of individual JAKs depends on their selective interactions with particular cytokine receptors. The JAK-STAT pathways downregulate more than 50 cytokines and growth factors and are considered a central communication node for the immune system.[1,2]

Many JAK inhibitors (JAKi) have been approved over the past few years by the US Food and Drug Administration/European Medicines Agency (FDA/EMA). Tofacitinib, a selective JAK1 and JAK3 inhibitor, has been approved for treating rheumatoid arthritis (RA), psoriatic arthritis, and ulcerative colitis. Ruxolitinib, a selective JAK1 and JAK2 inhibitor, has been approved for treating myelofibrosis and polycythemia vera. Baricitinib selectively inhibits JAK1 and JAK2 and has been approved for treating RA and atopic dermatitis (AD). Many newer JAKi used in dermatology have been listed in **Table 1**.[2,3] JAKi have been approved in alopecia areata (AA), vitiligo, psoriatic arthritis, chronic pruritic dermatoses including hand eczemas, and AD.

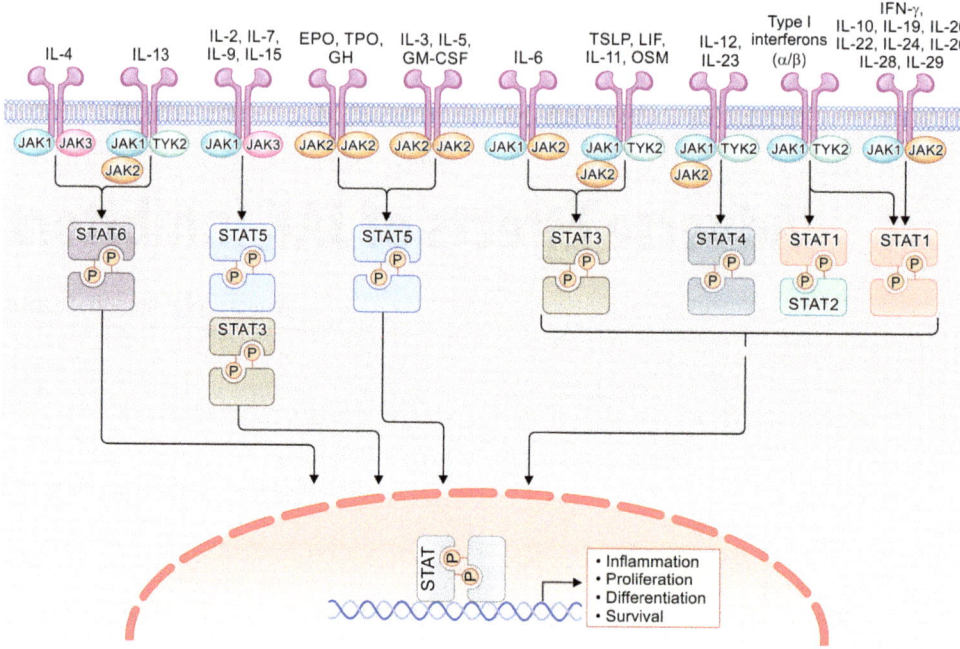

(EPO: erythropoietin; GM-CSF: granulocyte-macrophage colony-stimulating factor; GH: growth hormone; IL: interleukin; IFN-γ: interferon gamma; JAK: Janus kinase; LIF: leukemia inhibitory factor; OSM: oncostatin M; STAT: signal transducer and activator of transcription; TPO: thrombopoietin; TSLP: thymic stromal lymphopoietin)

FIG. 1: Types of JAK receptors and their mechanism of action.

TABLE 1	List of JAKi approved in dermatological conditions and their site of action.						
Drugs	JAK1-JAK3	JAK1-JAK2	JAK2-JAK2	TYK2-JAK2	TYK2-JAK1	JAK2-JAK1	FDA approval
Tofacitinib *JAK1, 2, 3 inhibitor*	+	+	+	+	+	+	• Psoriatic arthritis • Rheumatoid arthritis • Ulcerative colitis
Ruxolitinib *JAK1, 2 inhibitor*	+	+	+	+	+	+	• Rheumatoid arthritis • Polycythemia vera • Mycosis fungoides • Atopic dermatitis • Vitiligo and GVHD
Baricitinib *JAK1, 2 inhibitor*	+	+	+	+	+	+	• Rheumatoid arthritis • Alopecia areata • Atopic dermatitis
Upadacitinib *JAK1 inhibitor*	+	+	−	−	+	−	• Psoriatic arthritis • Rheumatoid arthritis • Deucrava • Ulcerative colitis • Alopecia areata • Ankylosing spondylitis
Abrocitinib *JAK1 inhibitor*	+	+	−	−	+	−	Atopic dermatitis

(JAKi: Janus kinase inhibitor; FDA: Food and Drug Administration; GVHD: graft-versus-host disease; TYK: tyrosine kinase)

■ ADVERSE EFFECTS

The list of adverse effects of JAKi is ever evolving. Since tofacitinib was the first JAKi to be used, it makes up for > 90% of the total number of adverse events reported due to JAKi.[4,5]

Female patients accounted for approximately 74–86% of those reporting adverse events in different studies. 45% of adverse events were reported above the age of 60 years.[5]

What is the reason for adverse events?
With the increased use of this class of drugs it is important to understand the possible cause of adverse events. The different members of the JAK family, JAK1, JAK2, JAK3, and TYK2, exhibit unique expression patterns in varied cell types. As they mediate actions of cytokines, (**Fig. 1 and Table 2**) inhibition would lead to side effects, but notably the inhibition is not absolute and is dose and site dependent, which accounts for the largely safe profile of these drugs in clinical practice (**Fig. 2**).

It is important to know the normal expression and biological function of the varied JAK receptors. *JAK1* serves as a central mediator in multiple cytokine signaling pathways, including class II, γc receptor, and gp130 subunit receptors and thus would affect the immune responses, antitumor immunity, and bone homeostasis, which is the reason it is used for selective intervention. *JAK2* is primarily activated by erythropoietin, interleukin 3 (IL-3), and granulocyte-macrophage colony-stimulating factor (GM-CSF), and is essential for erythropoiesis, thrombopoiesis, and granulocyte differentiation. *JAK3* is indispensable for lymphoid functions and hematopoietic cell differentiation, modulating proinflammatory cytokine production in innate immune cells. While JAK1 and JAK2 are broadly expressed, JAK3 is confined to hematopoietic cells and lymphoid tissues. Thus inhibition of JAK3 would lead lymphopenia and as JAK3 mediate cytokines that prevent infection, its use would also predispose to infections. TYK2, in contrast, is found in both immune and nonimmune cells. JAK expression varies among immune cell types, reflecting their specific roles in signaling and functions (**Table 1**).

Infections associated with JAKi are due to mechanisms related to the blockade of cytokines that use JAK-STAT for signaling pathways required for the host defense, leading to serious and/or opportunistic infections, such as herpes zoster (HZ).[1,6] The exact cause of *thromboembolic* events is not certain. Theoretically, inhibition of JAK should result in reduction of both autoimmune diseases' activity and reduction of prothrombotic risk. The process of thrombopoietin signaling and cancer immunoediting might be due to a variety of cytokines, such as interferon gamma and cell types such as NK cell, which could be affected by JAK inhibition.[5] Thromboembolic episodes (TEs) are believed to be due to specific JAK inhibition, where an antithrombotic pathway is blocked, while other pathways

TABLE 2	Overview of cytokines, JAK receptors, and the side effect profile.	
Ligands/Cytokines	**JAK**	**Side effects**
IL-2, IL-4, IL-6, IL-7, IL-9, IL-11, IL-10, IL-15, IFN-α, IFN-β, IFN-γ	JAK1	Immune suppression, hyperlipidemia
EPO, TPO, GM-CSF, IL-3, IL-5, IFN-γ	JAK2	Anemia, neutropenia, thrombocytopenia
IL-2, IL-4, IL-7, IL-9, IL-15	JAK3	Immune suppression
IFN-α, IFN-β, IFN-γ, IL-12	TYK2	Immune suppression
Immunoglobulins	SYK	Immune suppression

(EPO: erythropoietin; GM-CSF: granulocyte-macrophage colony-stimulating factor; IFN: interferon; IL: interleukin; JAK: Janus kinase; SYK: spleen tyrosine kinase; TPO: thrombopoietin; TYK: tyrosine kinase)

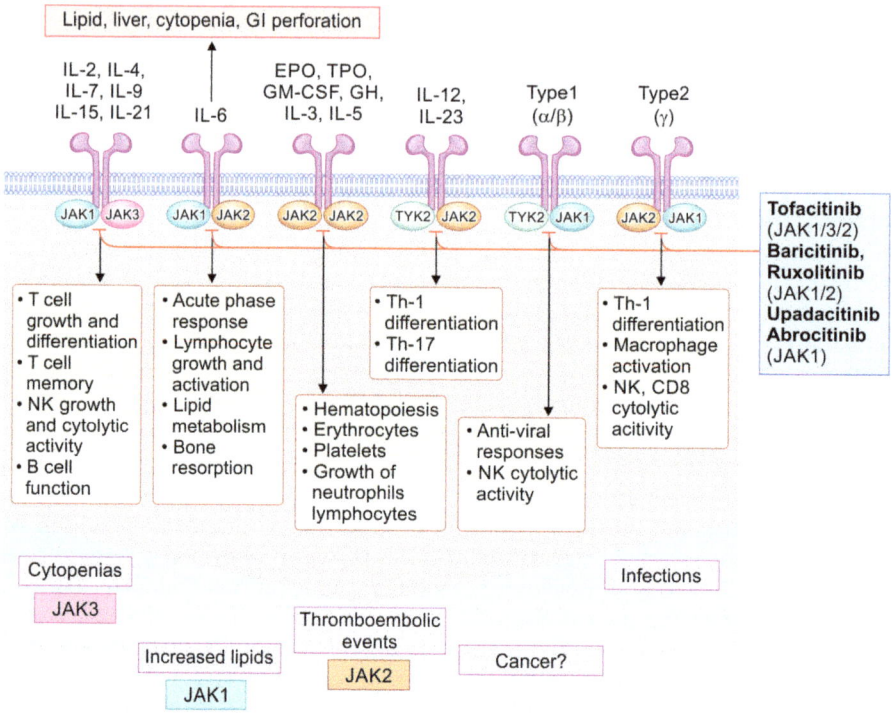

FIG. 2: Mechanism of adverse effects of JAK inhibitors.

(EPO: erythropoietin; GM-CSF: granulocyte-macrophage colony-stimulating factor; GH: growth hormone; IL: interleukin; JAK: Janus kinase; LIF: leukemia inhibitory factor; NK: natural killer; TPO: thrombopoietin)

that can transmit prothrombotic signals are not affected.[7] Notably in September 2021, FDA issued a black box warning about an increased risk of serious heart-related events, such as heart attack or stroke, cancer, blood clots, and death in patients treated with JAKi used for RA and ulcerative colitis.[8] It must be noted that this was noted in a population of RA with concomitant oral glucocorticosteroids and if the risk factors of venous thromboembolism (VTE) are excluded in routine practice, this is not commonly encountered. In fact, this is another reason for not combining oral steroids with JAKi.

The pathogenic pathways of *malignancy* due to JAKi are possibly due to varied mechanisms. Multiple pathways are likely to contribute to cancer risk in people on immunosuppressive medications, and risks may vary according to cancer type. For example, tofacitinib prevents natural killer (NK) cell maturation and tumor lysis capacity, which play important roles in anticancer immunosurveillance. Some treatments may lower the risk of certain cancers (e.g., lymphoma) through improved disease control, while increasing the risk of other cancers linked to immunosuppression [e.g., nonmelanoma skin cancer (NMSC)].[9] Nevertheless, since most JAKi, expect tofacitinib, have been used for a short period after marketing, and have a theoretical risk, it is necessary for a continuous pharmacovigilance on these adverse events. For now except for screening for NMSC once a year, there is no other advice with long-term usage.

While we will detail the varied side effects, an overview is provided in **Table 3** as a ready reckoner. It is important to mention here that tofacitinib has been safely used for more than 9.5 years in RA as per existing literature and thus the clinician does not need to be overtly alarmed by the iteration of adverse events.

TABLE 3	Common adverse events with JAKi.
Infections	• *Cause*: Due to the inhibitory effect on varied cytokines like IFN-γ and possibly muting the effect of TNF • Reactivation of varicella zoster virus if JAKi are used with steroids and MTX (risk factors: Age, female, steroids, > 20 mg). In India must rule out TB
Lymphopenia and hematologic alterations	*Cause*: The JAK1/3 receptors mediate lymphocyte development and host immune response. JAK2 receptors regulate hematopoietic cell development
Thromboembolic events	• *Cause*: Exact reason not known • ↑*Risk*: Age (>65 years), obesity, immobility, hereditary, COX2, prednisolone ≥ 7.5 mg/day, major surgery, ↑10 mg BD (tofacitinib), and baseline CVS risk
Dyslipidemia	• *Cause*: Related to targeting of IL-6 • Tofacitinib given as monotherapy, cause ↑LDL, HDL, and total cholesterol
Liver functions	Usually mild increase in enzymes, but there can be major derangements, especially with previously prescribe hepatotoxic agents
Malignancies	NMSC followed by lung cancer and lymphoma
Other*	• *Musculoskeletal*: Arthralgia, stiffness, Joint swelling, back pain, fibromyalgia, myalgia, and muscle fatigue • Varied other adverse events have been reported and are minor in nature related to the ocular, respiratory, psychiatric, cardiac, renal, endocrine, and metabolic aspects

*Tofacitinib

(COX2: cyclooxygenase-2; CVS: cardiovascular system; HDL: high-density lipoprotein; IFN: interferon; IL: interleukin; JAKi: Janus kinase inhibitor; LDL: low-density lipoprotein; NMSC: nonmelanoma skin cancer; TNF: tumor necrosis factor; TB: tuberculosis)

Source: Sardana K. Systemic Drugs in Dermatology, JAK inhibitors. Jaypee brothers; Ch 7. p. 503.

TABLE 4	Overview of salient Janus kinase (JAK)-specific adverse events.
Tofacitinib	Infections, malignancies, anemia, neutropenia, elevated serum creatinine and transaminases, hypercholesterolemia, gastrointestinal symptoms, and thromboembolism
Ruxolitinib	Infections, malignancies, elevated creatinine kinase, elevated creatinine, and hyperlipidemia
Baricitinib	Infections, malignancies, and hyperlipidemia
Delgocitinib	Nasopharyngitis, Kaposi's varicella, contact dermatitis, and acne
Upadacitinib	Infections, malignancies, elevated lipid parameters, increased creatinine phosphokinase, increased hepatic aminotransferase, low blood cell counts, stroke, and venous thromboembolisms
Abrocitinib	Nasopharyngitis, nausea, vomiting, acne, herpes zoster, increased blood creatinine phosphokinase, dizziness, and headache
Deucravacitinib	Nasopharyngitis and upper respiratory tract infections

Certain adverse events are specific to certain JAKi and are detailed in **Table 4**, but they again mirror largely the cytokine inhibition.

We will now discuss the varied systemic and dermatological side effects of JAKi.

SYSTEMIC SIDE EFFECTS OF JANUS KINASE INHIBITORS

A large database that analyzed 376,487 adverse events[3] found that four main organ classes were affected: "infections and infestations", "musculoskeletal and connective tissue disorders", "investigations", and "neoplasms benign, malignant and unspecified" (**Fig. 3**). The other systems affected included blood and lymphatic system and respiratory, thoracic, and mediastinal disorders, and we will attempt at discussing these aspects further. The systemic side effects are divided into:
- Treatment-emergent adverse events (TEAE)
- Serious adverse event (SAE)
- Common adverse events

Treatment Emergent Adverse Events

Treatment-emergent adverse events is defined as "an event that emerges during treatment, having been absent pretreatment, or worsens relative to the pretreatment state" according to the International Council for Harmonisation (ICH) E9 guideline.[10]

Infections and infestations represent the most common TEAE by MedDRA system organ class (SOC). A study conducted by Cohen et al. spanning 9.5 years of cumulative tofacitinib exposure in >7,000 patients, and representing the largest clinical dataset for a JAKi in RA showed that the **four** most common TEAEs were viral upper respiratory tract infection (URTI) (17.3%), URTI (17.2%), urinary tract infection (11.8%), and bronchitis (11.3%).[11]

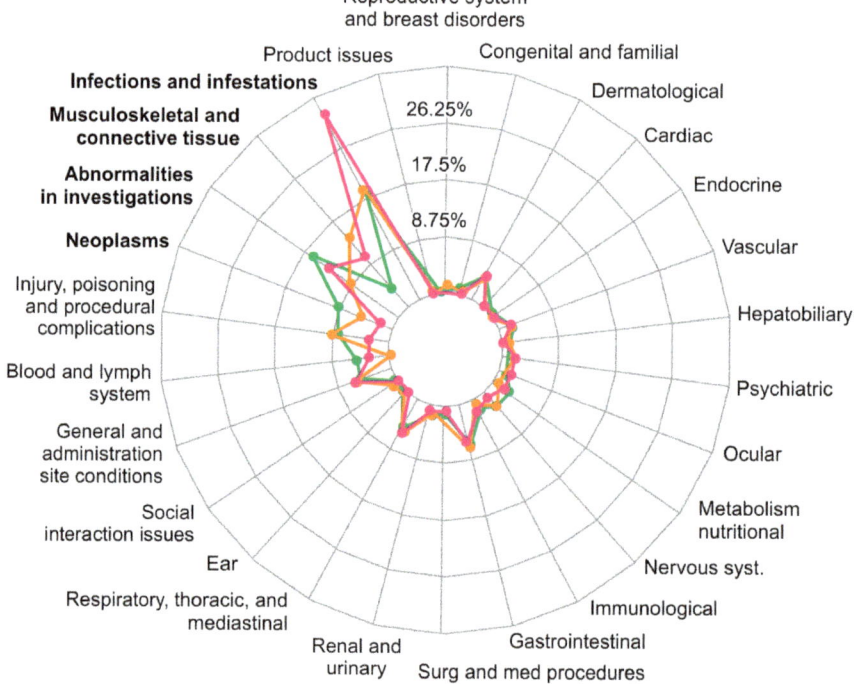

FIG. 3: The proportions of side effects of three JAK inhibitors as per organ system involvement. Orange curve represents tofacitinib, pink represents baricitinib and green represents ruxolitinib.

Source: Adapted from Hoisnard L, Lebrun-Vignes B, Maury S, Mahevas M, El Karoui K, Roy L, et al. Adverse events associated with JAK inhibitors in 126,815 reports from the WHO pharmacovigilance database. Sci Rep. 2022;12:7140.

Serious Adverse Events

Serious adverse events include:
- Serious infections
- Thromboembolic events
- Major adverse cardiovascular events (MACE), which included cardiovascular (CV) death, nonfatal myocardial infarction, and stroke
- Malignancy

Serious Infections

In AD patients on JAKi: The rates of serious infections in the JADE trials with abrocitinib ranged from 0.8 to 1.9% for abrocitinib 100/200 mg. The infections reported were herpangina and pneumonia, but the difference between the treatment group and the placebo was not significant.[12] Among patients receiving upadacitinib 15 or 30 mg the rates of serious infections ranged from 0.4 to 2.6% and included pneumonia and eczema herpeticum.[13]

In AA patients on JAKi: The incidence of serious infections in the baricitinib-treated patients of AA was 0–1.4% (2/4 mg) and included coronavirus disease 2019 (COVID-19), pneumonia, and pyelonephritis.[14]

In psoriasis patients on JAKi: Rates of serious infections were 1.1–2% in deucravacitinib with community-acquired pneumonia being the most common serious infection (0.3%).[2]

In RA patients treated with JAKi: Serious adverse infections which required hospitalization occurred in 8.2% RA patients treated with tofacitinib. The most common SAEs were pneumonia ($n = 124$), HZ ($n = 43$), urinary tract infection ($n = 31$), and cellulitis ($n = 31$). The incidence rates of SAEs gradually decreased over time with longer exposure to tofacitinib.[11]

Major Adverse Cardiovascular Events

It has been noted that no MACE have been reported with higher reporting for JAKi. Similarly, no cerebrovascular events were reported with JAKi. Nevertheless, it is important to know which patient subset is prone to MACE. Thus, this is higher in patients with RA with a history of atherosclerotic CV disease (i.e., coronary artery disease, cerebrovascular disease, or peripheral artery disease), compared with patients without a history of atherosclerotic CV disease.

In AD patients on JAKi: Sudden cardiac death (aortic valve sclerosis and untreated hypertension) was reported in one patient (0.6%) on abrocitinib. Similarly one patient (0.1%) on upadacitinib had a myocardial infarction related to coronavirus disease.[2,12]

In AA patients on JAKi: Phase 3 trials on baricitinib reported one patient (0.5%) who had pre-existent comorbidities and suffered from myocardial infarction.[14] A meta-analysis of five randomized controlled trials (RCTs) of AA on JAKi reported severe or life-threatening events in 0.3%, which included two cases of rhabdomyolysis (brepocitinib), one case of myocardial infarction (baricitinib), and one case of hypertensive urgency (tofacitinib).[8]

In vitiligo patients on JAKi: Phase 3 trials of ruxolitinib cream in vitiligo reported 2 out of 637 developing myocarditis and coronary artery stenosis, which were found to be unrelated to treatment.[2,15]

In psoriasis patients on JAKi: The rates of MACE were 0.2–0.4% in deucravacitinib treated patients and included non-ST elevation myocardial infarction and cerebrovascular accident.[2]

Thromboembolic Events

Among the 126,815 adverse events reported in the World Health Organization (WHO) pharmacovigilance database, 1,803 (1.4%) described embolism and thrombosis. Thromboembolic adverse events were ranked from the *highest* for *baricitinib*, then ruxolitinib and then tofacitinib.[3]

In RA patients treated with JAKi: VTE [i.e., deep vein thrombosis (DVT) and/or pulmonary embolism (PE)] was reported in 59 (0.8%) patients, while arterial thromboembolism was reported in 84 (1.2%) patients. The reporting odds ratio of PE was disproportionately high with baricitinib, as was the risk of DVT.[5] A recent Swedish study reported that baricitinib and tofacitinib are associated with a 50–100% increased risk of PE compared with biological disease-modifying antirheumatic drugs (bDMARDs).[16]

In AD patients on JAKi: The rates of TE were found to be rare, ranging from 0 to 0.5% in phase 3 trials of abrocitinib with one patient having a nonfatal retinal vein thrombosis, leading to discontinuation of abrocitinib, while 2/1,608 (0.1%) patients had a TE in upadacitinib-treated groups. Both the events were found to be unrelated to therapy.[13,17] A meta-analysis of two cohort studies and 15 RCTs with a total of 466,993 participants concluded that patients with AD on JAKi *did not* have an increased risk of VTE.[18]

In AA patients on JAKi: In the existing literature, there are no described cases of TE in AA patients on baricitinib.[2]

In psoriasis patients on JAKi: The rates of TE in deucravacitinib-treated patients were 1/531 (0.2%) and 1/833 (0.1%). One had pulmonary artery thrombosis and other radial artery thrombosis.[2]

The **risk factors** associated with an increased risk of TE events are:
- Age ≥ 50 years
- Patients with baseline CV risk factors—current smoker
- High-density lipoprotein level < 40 mg/dL
- History of hypertension
- Diabetes
- Myocardial infarction or coronary heart disease
- Patients with uncontrolled, high immune-mediated disease activity
- High dose of tofacitinib (> 20 mg)

Needless to say that incidence rates in patients *without risk factors* were very *low*[3] and conversely in case of risk factors, probably these drugs should be avoided for long-term use.

Malignancy

The WHO database have shown that "hematopoietic neoplasms (excluding leukemias and lymphomas)", "skin neoplasms malignant and unspecified", "leukemias" and "soft tissue neoplasms benign", and "respiratory and mediastinal neoplasms malignant" have been reported. But extrapolating data from rheumatology, there is no significant increase except for NMSC, which might be elevated and thus regular skin examinations, is important, especially in countries with increased risk of NMSC, such as Australia. While current malignancy (except NMSC and cervical carcinoma in situ undergoing treatment) may be a contraindication for JAKi, but as stated previously, this should be a shared decision making with the patient.

In AD patients on JAKi: There are no reported events of NMSC and non-NMSC malignancy in the abrocitinib phase 3 trials. NMSC was the most reported malignancy occurring in 0.5% patients on upadacitinib 15 and 30 mg. In a total of 1,608 patients treated with upadacitinib, other non-NMSC malignancies were noted: breast cancer ($n = 1$), gastric cancer ($n = 1$), and anal cancer.[2]

In AA patients on JAKi: The incidence of malignancy was 0/183 and 1/155 (0.6%) in AA patients compared with 1/154 (0.6%) in placebo. One baricitinib-treated patient developed B-cell lymphoma, and one receiving placebo had prostate cancer.[2]

In psoriasis patients on JAKi: Rates of NMSC were 0.4–0.9% among deucravacitinib-treated patients compared with no events in the placebo. The malignancies reported are basal cell carcinoma and squamous cell carcinoma in the deucravacitinib group. Rates of non-NMSC were 0.2–0.4% in deucravacitinib compared with no events in the placebo. The reported cases were: Hodgkin's lymphoma ($n = 1$), breast cancer ($n = 1$), and hepatocellular carcinoma ($n = 1$) and are lower than the background rates previously reported in psoriasis in the Market Scan studies.[2]

In RA patients on JAKi: The most common malignancies related to exposure to tofacitinib were lung cancer, breast cancer, and lymphoma. The incidence rates of overall malignancy were 0.85 and 0.8 per 100 patient-years for tofacitinib and baricitinib, respectively.[19] In a network meta-analysis of 62 eligible RCTs and 16 long-term extension studies, with 82,366 person-years of exposure to JAKi, it was found that JAKi were associated with a higher incidence of malignancy compared with TNF inhibitor but not placebo or methotrexate.[9]

Common Adverse Effects

These include:
- Infections
- Gastrointestinal (GI) adverse events
- Neurological changes

Infections

As discussed previously JAKi can in theory diminish the host defense against pathogens. In RA population, the common infections were nasopharyngitis, upper respiratory infections, gastroenteritis, or bronchitis. Increased infection rates were observed in a systematic review investigating safety events, especially HZ, tuberculosis (TB), cellulitis, panniculitis, septic shock, and osteomyelitis.

In a recent study,[3] herpes viral infections were reported *highest* for *baricitinib*, followed by tofacitinib and ruxolitinib. Dose-dependent occurrence of herpes infection was noted with baricitinib. Influenza viral infections were reported maximally with tofacitinib followed by baricitinib and ruxolitinib.

Herpes zoster has been reported to be more frequent than bDMARDs and is especially frequent in Japan and Korea. Moreover, EMA (but not FDA) has restricted the use of tofacitinib in people older than 65 years due to an increased risk of serious infection.

Amongst fungal infectious disorders, pneumocystis infections, and cryptococcal and *Coccidioides* infections were common specifically pneumocystis infections, which was over-reported for baricitinib versus tofacitinib and ruxolitinib.[3]

The most common *organs* to be affected were—URTIs, urinary tract infections, and lower respiratory tract and lung infections.[3]

In RA patients on JAKi: Opportunistic infections other than TB were reported in 90 (1.3%) patients on tofacitinib 5 mg and 10 mg. Incidence rates were not related with increasing tofacitinib exposure. HZ was the most common infection (57 of 90 cases). There were five cases of cryptococcal infection.

The *risk factors* which significantly affected the risk of opportunistic infections were tofacitinib dose, higher age, geographical region, chronic obstructive pulmonary disease (COPD), and prior confirmed post-baseline lymphopenia < 1,000 cells/µL.[5,11]

In AD patients on JAKi: Herpes simplex was reported more frequently in patients with AD receiving upadacitinib (3.3–7.7%) compared with 1.7% in placebo than those on abrocitinib (0–2% in abrocitinib compared with 1.8% in placebo). No TB reactivation was seen with both the drugs.[2] Notably, the data from TB endemic countries may have a different conclusion.

In AA patients on JAKi: Common infections in baricitinib-treated patients included URTI and urinary tract infections. The URTI incidence was almost similar in the baricitinib and placebo groups. Urinary tract infection was reported in 4.7–7.7% in the baricitinib group. Herpes infection was more in the placebo group as compared to the baricitinib group (2.1 vs. 1.8%).[2]

In vitiligo patients on JAKi: Nasopharyngitis occurred in 4.4% in ruxolitinib-treated patients as compared to 0.9% in placebo.[2]

In psoriasis patients on JAKi: Rates of URTIs and nasopharyngitis were 21/322 (6.3%) each in deucravacitinib. HZ was uncommon, 1.2% of patients compared with none in the placebo.[2]

Tuberculosis and JAKi: A meta-analysis has shown that in RA patients treated with JAKi, the risk of TB was dose-dependent and was higher than placebo, but was not statistically significant. The incidence rate of TB was significantly correlated with the country's background incidence rates of TB.[20] The risk of TB was less with JAKi as compared to TNF-α inhibitors.[21] A large database of continuous use of tofacitinib for 9.5 years showed that latent TB was reported in 130 and 190 patients receiving tofacitinib 5 and 10 mg BID, respectively, which was adequately treated with prophylaxis.[11] Translating this to India, it is imperative to diagnose latent TB infection with a tuberculin skin test and/or interferon gamma release assay prior to starting JAKi. (See chapter on Baseline Tests and Monitoring)

Gastrointestinal Adverse Events

In AD patients on JAKi: The most common GI side effect was nausea and was reported in 14/156 (9%) with abrocitinib 100 mg, 31/154 (20%) with abrocitinib 200 mg.[1,2] Upadacitinib also showed a dosage-dependent increase in nausea ranging from 2.4 to 7.1%. Diarrhea was reported in 7% of patients on upadacitinib and abrocitinib.[2]

In AA patients on JAKi: GI disorders were not reported among the common adverse events in patients with AA receiving baricitinib.[2]

In psoriasis patients on JAKi: No difference was seen between the drug and placebo group with respect to nausea and diarrhea.[2]

In RA patients on JAKi: GI perforations were reported in 28 (0.4%) patients and mostly with tofacitinib. Lower GI tract was most commonly involved in perforations, and *all except two* occurred in patients with underlying risk factors. 26 patients received concomitant therapy with one or more nonsteroidal anti-inflammatory drugs (NSAIDs) or glucocorticoids.[2] 13 patients had at least one of the following underlying relevant diseases and/or surgeries:

history of gastric perforation with peritonitis, diverticulitis, irritable bowel syndrome, colon polyp, gastroenteritis, or gastric ulcer; current event of spastic colon, gastritis, gastroduodenitis or diverticulitis; and history of cholecystectomy and/or appendectomy with or without gastric ulcer.[5,11]

Neurological Side Effects[2]

In AD patients on JAKi: Headaches were the most common neurologic side effect and were reported in 8% in abrocitinib 100 mg group, 10% in 200 mg abrocitinib group,[4,5,7-9] 5% in patients on upadacitinib and 3% in placebo groups. The headaches were relatively short-lived with a mean duration of 4 days in the abrocitinib 100 mg group and 3 days in the 200 mg group.

In AA patients on JAKi: Headaches occurred in 4.4–9% of patients on baricitinib compared with 4.8–6.5% in placebo.

In vitiligo patients on JAKi: Headaches occurred in 2.7–4.8% compared with 1.8–3.5% in placebo.

In psoriasis patients on JAKi: Headaches had an incidence of 4.8% compared with 3% in placebo.

Laboratory Abnormalities

Laboratory abnormalities are without clinical sequelae in the majority of patients. The only adverse event on consequence is anemia, which is consequent to **JAK2 inhibition**, which is involved in **EPO signaling**. Cytopenias may occur but were not more frequent than on placebo, although with all JAKi a few patients may exhibit neutropenia and/or lymphopenia. While the topic of baseline tests and monitoring will be addressed in a separate chapter (see Chapter Baseline Tests and Monitoring), here we will dwell on the major abnormalities.

Complete Blood Count

A dose-related decrease in platelet count was noted at the end of the fourth week with abrocitinib, while transient neutropenia was noted with upadacitinib when given in patients with AD.[12] Transient anemia, neutropenia, and thrombocytosis was seen in isolated patients, which normalized while on treatment in patients given baricitinib for AA.[2]

Lipids

A dose-related elevation of approximately 10% in high- and low-density lipoprotein (HDL and LDL) cholesterol levels have been noted with abrocitinib. 40% increase in HDL and 25% increase in LDL was noted in patients on baricitinib for AA.[2] It must be noted that while increased levels may seem alarming, they do not impact on cardiovascular system (CVS) mortality and notably the changes in lipid levels may represent a response to attenuation of inflammation. In fact, there is a well-established "lipid paradox theory" which emphasizes the U-shaped relationship between LDL cholesterol and CV risk.

Creatinine Phosphokinase

This was the most common laboratory abnormality seen in patients of AD on JAKi. It was occasionally seen in patients with AA and psoriasis also.[2] While creatinine phosphokinase (CPK) elevations are occasionally seen without weakness, thus far with occasional myalgia, there are little clinical effects and unless guided by symptoms, there is no need to test for CPK.

Liver Function Test and Kidney Function Test

Slight elevations in serum creatinine rates have been observed across all JAKi studies but were not associated with nephropathic changes or a clinical correlate leading to end-stage renal disease. Slight elevations of transaminases have been observed for all the approved JAKi, except for filgotinib. Abnormalities resolved after reduction or discontinuation.

Dermatological Side Effects
Oral Janus Kinase Inhibitors[2]

In AD patients on oral JAKi: The most common dermatologic adverse events were acne and AD. With abrocitinib, acne was recorded in 2% of patients on the 100 mg dose and in 4.7–5.8% of patients on the 200 mg dose. It was reported in 1.5–3.6% of patients on upadacitinib. It was more frequent among younger, female, and non-white patients. The lesion responded with topical medications.

Atopic dermatitis was reported as a side effect in 14% of patients on abrocitinib 100 mg and in 5% of patients on the 200 mg dose versus 17% in the placebo. In comparison, 1% of patients in the upadacitinib 15 mg groups and 9% of patients in the 30 mg groups versus 3% in the placebo reported AD.

In AA patients on JAKi: Acne was more common in the baricitinib-treated groups than in the placebo.

In psoriasis patients on JAKi: Acne occurred in 2.8% in deucravacitinib compared with no events in placebo.

Topical Janus Kinase Inhibitors

Topical JAKi aim to improve drug delivery to the skin areas affected by the disease, accelerating the onset of action and reducing the risk of serious adverse drug reactions usually associated with oral formulations.[22] This premise does not hold true in clinical practice as the results of topical JAKi are inferior to oral drugs. Ruxolitinib was the first drug in this class to be approved and is indicated for mild to moderate AD and has been shown to lessen pruritus, reduce pain and eczema, and improve sleeping.[23]

Most of the data on adverse events with topical medication is limited and most of the adverse drug reactions associated with topical JAKi are expected, localized, and nonserious. Evidence suggests that patients with severe AD are at an increased risk of experiencing more severe adverse effects.

A network meta-analysis of 10 RCTs on topical JAKi comparing multiple treatment formulations in AD (tofacitinib, ruxolitinib, delgocitinib, topical triamcinolone, tacrolimus, and placebo) showed that:[23]

- *For any adverse events*: Topical tofacitinib has a reduced risk of adverse events as compared to ruxolitinib and also to topical tacrolimus.
- *For SAEs*: Topical triamcinolone acetonide (TAC) was the safest followed by delgocitinib and ruxolitinib.
- *For adverse events leading to treatment discontinuation*: The risk of adverse events leading to discontinuation is lower with every treatment than with placebo. Tofacitinib was the safest treatment, followed by delgocitinib and ruxolitinib.
- *For infections*: Topical TAC is associated with a lower risk of any infection than ruxolitinib. According to the ranking, TAC is the safest treatment, followed by placebo, tacrolimus, and JAKi.

- *For application site reactions*: All treatments present a reduced risk of any application-site reactions compared with placebo. Topical TAC was the safest treatment, followed by delgocitinib and ruxolitinib.

■ CONCLUSION

Janus kinase inhibitors mediate their action through various cytokines, the inhibition of which is believed to result in side effects. But contrary to what was believed the side effects are not common nor consistently seen. This is evident by the almost 10 years of use in rheumatological literature. The side effect profile of JAKi is ever changing and ranges from laboratory abnormalities without clinical sequelae to serious life-threatening complications. The available data shows that the incidence of the latter is very low and this is seen predominantly in patients with comorbid risk factors. Uncommon and serious life-threatening side effects should be reported.

The scope of JAKi in dermatology is expanding; therefore, it is vital to have a continuous pharmacovigilance on part of the treating dermatologist.[24]

■ REFERENCES

1. Tanaka Y, Luo Y, O'Shea JJ, Nakayamada S. Janus kinase-targeting therapies in rheumatology: a mechanisms-based approach. Nat Rev Rheumatol. 2022;18:133-45.
2. Samuel C, Cornman H, Kambala A, Kwatra SG. A Review on the Safety of Using JAK Inhibitors in Dermatology: Clinical and Laboratory Monitoring. Dermatol Ther (Heidelb). 2023;13:729-49.
3. Hoisnard L, Lebrun-Vignes B, Maury S, Mahevas M, El Karoui K, Roy L, et al. Adverse events associated with JAK inhibitors in 126,815 reports from the WHO pharmacovigilance database. Sci Rep. 2022;12:7140.
4. US FDA. FDA-approved Drugs. [online] Available from http://www.accessdata.fda.gov/scripts/cder/drugsatfda/ [Last accessed January, 2024].
5. Song YK, Song J, Kim K, Kwon JW. Potential Adverse Events Reported With the Janus Kinase Inhibitors Approved for the Treatment of Rheumatoid Arthritis Using Spontaneous Reports and Online Patient Reviews. Front Pharmacol. 2022;12:792877.
6. Adas MA, Alveyn E, Cook E, Dey M, Galloway JB, Bechman K. The infection risks of JAK inhibition. Expert Rev Clin Immunol. 2022;18:253-61.
7. Kotyla PJ, Engelmann M, Giemza-Stokłosa J, Wnuk B, Islam MA. Thromboembolic Adverse Drug Reactions in Janus Kinase (JAK) Inhibitors: Does the Inhibitor Specificity Play a Role? Int J Mol Sci. 2021;22:2449.
8. Sechi A, Song J, Dell'Antonia M, Heidemeyer K, Piraccini BM, Starace M, et al. Adverse events in patients treated with Jak-inhibitors for alopecia areata: A systematic review. J Eur Acad Dermatol Venereol. 2023. [Online ahead of print].
9. Russell MD, Stovin C, Alveyn E, Adeyemi O, Chan CKD, Patel V, et al. JAK inhibitors and the risk of malignancy: a meta-analysis across disease indications. Ann Rheum Dis. 2023;82(8):1059-67.
10. Nilsson ME, Koke SC. Defining Treatment-Emergent Adverse Events with the Medical Dictionary for Regulatory Activities (MedDRA). Ther Innov Regul Sci. 2001;35:1289-99.
11. Cohen SB, Tanaka Y, Mariette X, Curtis JR, Lee EB, Nash P, et al. Long-term safety of tofacitinib up to 9.5 years: a comprehensive integrated analysis of the rheumatoid arthritis clinical development programme. RMD Open. 2020;6:e001395.
12. Simpson EL, Sinclair R, Forman S, Wollenberg A, Aschoff R, Cork M, et al. Efficacy and safety of abrocitinib in adults and adolescents with moderate-to-severe atopic dermatitis (JADE MONO-1): a multicentre, double-blind, randomised, placebo-controlled, phase 3 trial. Lancet. 2020;396(10246):255-66.
13. Simpson EL, Papp KA, Blauvelt A, Chu CY, Hong HC, Katoh N, et al. Efficacy and safety of upadacitinib in patients with moderate to severe atopic dermatitis: analysis of follow-up data from the measure up 1 and measure up 2 randomized clinical trials. JAMA Dermatol. 2022;158:404-13.

14. King B, Ohyama M, Kwon O, Zlotogorski A, Ko J, Mesinkovska NA, et al. Two phase 3 trials of baricitinib for alopecia areata. N Engl J Med. 2022;386:1687-99.
15. Rosmarin D, Passeron T, Pandya AG, Grimes P, Harris JE, Desai SR, et al. Two phase 3, randomized, controlled trials of ruxolitinib cream for vitiligo. N Engl J Med. 2022;387:1445-55.
16. Molander V, Bower H, Frisell T, Delcoigne B, Di Giuseppe D, Askling J; The ARTIS study group. Venous thromboembolism with JAK inhibitors and other immune-modulatory drugs: a Swedish comparative safety study among patients with rheumatoid arthritis. Ann Rheum Dis. 2023;82:189-97.
17. Blauvelt A, Silverberg JI, Lynde CW, Bieber T, Eisman S, Zdybski J, et al. Abrocitinib induction, randomized withdrawal, and retreatment in patients with moderate-to-severe atopic dermatitis: Results from the JAK1 Atopic Dermatitis Efficacy and Safety (JADE) REGIMEN phase 3 trial. J Am Acad Dermatol. 2022;86(1):104-12.
18. Chen TL, Lee LL, Huang HK, Chen LY, Loh CH, Chi CC. Association of risk of incident venous thromboembolism with atopic dermatitis and treatment with Janus kinase inhibitors: a systematic review and meta-analysis. JAMA Dermatol. 2022;158(11):1254-61.
19. Harigai M. Growing Evidence of the Safety of JAK Inhibitors in Patients with Rheumatoid Arthritis. Rheumatology (Oxford). 2019;58(1):i34-i42.
20. Ji X, Hu L, Wang Y, Man S, Liu X, Song C, et al. Risk of tuberculosis in patients with rheumatoid arthritis treated with biological and targeted drugs: meta-analysis of randomized clinical trials. Chinese Med J. 2022;135:409-15.
21. Matsumoto T. Impact of Biologic and JAK Inhibitor Therapies on TB: How Do Biologic Therapies Affect the Presentation and Treatment Course of Pulmonary TB? In: Saito T, Narita M, Daley CL (Eds). Pulmonary Tuberculosis and Its Prevention. Respiratory Disease Series: Diagnostic Tools and Disease Managements. Singapore: Springer; 2022.
22. Papp K, Szepietowski JC, Kircik L, Toth D, Eichenfield LF, Leung DYM, et al. Efficacy and safety of ruxolitinib cream for the treatment of atopic dermatitis: results from 2 phase 3, randomized, double-blind studies. J Am Acad Dermatol. 2021;85(4):863-72.
23. Alves C, Penedones A, Mendes D, Batel Marques F. Topical Janus kinase inhibitors in atopic dermatitis: a safety network meta-analysis. Int J Clin Pharm. 2023;45:830-8.
24. Muddebihal A, Khurana A, Sardana K. JAK inhibitors in dermatology: the road travelled and path ahead, a narrative review. Expert Rev Clin Pharmacol. 2023;16(4):279-95.

CHAPTER 12

Baseline Tests and Monitoring

Ananta Khurana

"What gets monitored gets improved."
—Peter F Drucker

Overview

- Introduction
- Important Points to Note when Assessing Patient for Janus Kinase Inhibitor Use
- Baseline Testing
- Follow-up Monitoring

■ INTRODUCTION

With ever expanding use of Janus kinase inhibitors (JAKis),[1] a cautious watch must be kept for all possible adverse events. Although JAKis have favorable safety profiles, careful monitoring is essential, especially in certain high-risk groups. These are listed in **Box 1** and further detailed in the section below.

BOX 1 Scenarios where cautious use of JAKi is advised.

- Age > 65 years, BMI ≥ 30 kg/m², hypertension, heavy smoking, use of oral contraceptives, immobility, and steroids (risk factors for thromboembolism)
- History of previous thromboembolic episode; hereditary or acquired coagulation disorder
- History of tuberculosis
- Cardiac disease
- Severe renal or hepatic dysfunction
- Active hepatitis B and C infection
- Immunocompromised patients and those concomitantly on other immunosuppressive drugs (especially oral steroids)
- Pregnant and lactating women; women contemplating pregnancy
- Ongoing severe infection; history of a serious or an opportunistic infection; underlying conditions that may predispose a patient to infections
- Patients at increased risk of gastrointestinal perforations (patients with a history of diverticulitis and taking concomitant NSAIDs or glucocorticoids)

(BMI: body mass index; JAKi: Janus kinase inhibitor; NSAIDs: nonsteroidal anti-inflammatory drugs)

■ IMPORTANT POINTS TO NOTE WHEN ASSESSING PATIENT FOR JANUS KINASE INHIBITOR USE (BOX 1)[2-4]

- Janus kinase inhibitor has a **short-half-life**, but a gap of 4 weeks is recommended if a patient wants to conceive. In animal studies, tofacitinib was teratogenic and feticidal when used at doses several times higher than those used in humans. No fetal deaths or congenital malformations were observed in the clinical development programs for rheumatoid arthritis (RA), psoriasis, or inflammatory bowel disease.
- It is not known if the drugs are secreted in **human milk**, but in view of known secretion in animal studies, the use of JAKi is not recommended in lactating females.
- The risk of **thromboembolism** is mainly in patients with a previous history of thromboembolic events, those on hormone replacement therapy, those with other cardiovascular risk factors and advanced age and on high doses of JAKi (tofacitinib 20 mg/day) (also see Chapter 11).
- **Major cardiovascular adverse events** have been reported mainly in older patients, those who are current or past smokers and have other cardiovascular risk factors. JAKis should be discontinued in patients who experience a myocardial infarction or stroke.
- JAKis should not be used in presence of **severe hepatic disease** (Child-Pugh C). Dosage adjustment of tofacitinib is recommended in patients with moderate hepatic impairment, while no dosage adjustment is required in mild hepatic impairment. No dose adjustment is necessary however for baricitinib's use in patients with mild or moderate hepatic impairment.
- In presence of **severe renal disease** [creatinine clearance (CrCl) < 30 mL/min]: Reduce tofacitinib dose to 5 mg once daily, while baricitinib is not recommended at this level of renal dysfunction. With CrCl 30–60 mL/min, baricitinib should be used at 1 mg daily and at CrCl 60–< 90 mL/min at the dose of 2 mg/day. Abrocitinib's use is not recommended in presence of severe renal dysfunction (CrCL < 30 mL/min). A dose reduction to 50 mg/day is recommended with CrCl 30–60 mL/min, while a dose of 100 mg/day can be used for CrCL 60–90 mL/min.
- In patients with an **underlying malignancy**, it is advisable to take decision in consultation with the treating oncologist. Thus far, patient registries and clinical trial data have demonstrated no malignancy signal. There are no data to suggest that prior malignancy is problematic with JAKi therapy, but most studies excluded patients with malignant disease up to 5 years prior to enrolment.
- Consider **drug interactions** when starting: Tofacitinib is metabolized by cytochrome P450 (CYP450) pathway, and hence the simultaneous use of known promoters and inhibitors of the enzyme must be recorded. Importantly, when treating for latent tuberculosis infection (LTBI), isoniazid alone is preferable as rifampicin increases hepatic metabolism of tofacitinib. Upadacitinib and baricitinib are also mainly metabolized by CYP3A4, while for abrocitinib, oxidative metabolism is the primary route of elimination and use with strong inducers or inhibitors of CYP2C9 is to be avoided.
- The safety and efficacy of JAKi is under investigation in **juvenile patients** and has not yet been established for most JAKis in persons <18 years of age.
- Finally, JAKi have not been studied and therefore are not recommended in **combination** with biological disease-modifying antirheumatic drugs (bDMARDs) or potent **immunosuppressive agents** such as cyclosporine or tacrolimus because of the possibility of increased immunosuppression and increased risk of infection or lymphoma. Use with oral steroids leads to increased incidence of adverse effects, without significant addition in efficacy.

BASELINE TESTING

After it has been established that one is dealing with a condition potentially treatable with a JAKi, and possible risk factors have been assessed, a battery of baseline tests is recommended before commencing treatment.[5,6] The rationale is to elicit the underlying conditions which may form a contraindication to the use of JAKi or may need to be simultaneously managed if JAKi is initiated.

It is important to mention here the need for a baseline assessment (patient history followed by laboratory investigations as mentioned later) for tuberculosis prior to initiating JAKis, as India is a TB endemic country and reactivation of latent tuberculosis infection (LTBI) with JAKi has mostly been reported in geographical regions with a high prevalence of TB.

The baseline testing panel broadly includes the following:
- A complete blood count including absolute lymphocyte counts and absolute neutrophil counts
- Liver function testing
- Kidney function tests
- Lipid profile
- Hepatitis profile (hepatitis B surface antigen, antihepatitis C antibodies)
- Human immunodeficiency virus (HIV)
- A workup for active or latent tuberculosis: Chest X-ray, Mantoux test/interferon gamma release assays (IGRA)
- Additional tests: Creatine phosphokinase (for baricitinib)

Avoid commencing treatment with a JAKi in case any of the following is detected therapy should be witheld:
- Hemoglobin <9 g/dL, (<8 g/dL for abrocitinib and baricitinib)
- Absolute neutrophil counts <1,000/mm^3
- Absolute lymphocyte count <500/mm^3
- Additionally, abrocitinib should be avoided in presence of platelet counts <150,000/mm^3

The following conditions need further attention before commencing treatment:[7-15]

Latent TB infection (LTBI):[8,10] Screening for, and treatment of, LTBI (if detected) is an essential component of baseline investigations for initiating JAKis in high endemic areas, such as India. A reactivation of TB with JAKi may develop in lungs or an extrapulmonary site.

In resource poor settings, a Mantoux level of >10 mm in an adult indicates presence of LTBI (in high endemic areas), although various inconsistencies of Mantoux testing (site reading inaccuracies, false positivity with nontuberculous mycobacterial infection) should be kept in mind. Bacillus Calmette–Guérin (BCG) vaccination can also be a cause for a positive Mantoux test. Interferon gamma release assays (IGRA) overcome these inconsistencies and are preferable, if feasible, for baseline assessment. As a general rule, a positive Mantoux needs to be validated by IGRA.

Treatment for LTBI should ideally be initiated before starting JAKi (for 3 months), but in clinical situations both would often be started together. Isoniazid prophylaxis is preferable over isoniazid + rifampicin prophylaxis in patients on tofacitinib owing to significant pharmacokinetic interactions of tofacitinib with rifampicin (resulting in 80% reduction in bioavailability of tofacitinib). The same interaction has however not been observed with baricitinib even though in vitro studies suggest that baricitinib is a CYP3A4 substrate.

The risk of clinically significant hepatitis with combination of tofacitinib and isoniazid is extremely low. It is important to note that TB reactivation has been reported even in patients who tested negative at initial screening and in patients on continued treatment beyond the completion of LTBI prophylaxis. Hence, continued close watch is essential throughout the duration of JAKi treatment. A higher dose of tofacitinib 10 mg BD has been (inconsistently) shown to be associated with a greater risk of TB reactivation.

Hepatitis B and C infection: There is limited literature on reactivation of hepatitis B and C on JAKi. In a series of 98 RA patients, Ji et al. (2021)[13] reported that tofacitinib could induce hepatitis B virus (HBV) reactivation in both hepatitis B surface antigen+ (HBsAg+) and HBsAg-/HBcAb+ (core antibody +) RA patients. HBsAg+ patients receiving tofacitinib had a high incidence rate of HBV reactivation. The HBV reactivation rate was 33.3% in the HBsAg+ RA patients without antiviral prophylaxis and 3.1% in HBsAg-/HBcAb+ patients. Reactivation can however be prevented by antiviral prophylaxis and no patient on antiviral prophylaxis developed a reactivation. Thus, a hepatologist consult is essential prior to starting treatment with JAKi in such a scenario. The authors recommended that although the risk of reactivation is low in **HBsAg-/HBcAb+** patients, closely monitoring of HBV DNA and alanine aminotransferase should be suggested. In another series, no case of hepatitis B reactivation was noted amongst patients with resolved hepatitis B infection treated with tofacitinib (Serling et al.).[9]

There is much less literature on hepatitis C reactivation on JAKis. Chen et al. reported no increase in hepatitis C viral load in HCV-positive RA patients treated with tofacitinib for up to a year, without antiviral prophylaxis.[16]

HIV infection: JAKis (especially ruxolitinib and baricitinib) are being explored for a potential role in inhibiting HIV replication, reducing HIV reservoir and viral persistence, and in suppressing HIV-associated chronic inflammation.[17,18] In a recent randomized controlled trial (RCT) of healthy, virologically suppressed patients on antiretroviral therapy (ART), ruxolitinib was well tolerated and significantly decreased markers of immune activation and cell survival (Marconi 2022).[18] However, yet there are limited clinical reports on safe use of JAKis for other indications in known HIV patients (Hoff 2020), and cautious use is recommended.[19]

Vaccines: It is recommended to complete all age-appropriate vaccinations as recommended by current national immunization guidelines prior to starting JAKis. This mainly concerns use in small children. Avoid use of live vaccines just prior to, during, or just after treatment with JAKis.

■ FOLLOW-UP MONITORING

Regular assessment of the condition under treatment is essential and drug discontinuation should be contemplated once desired outcomes are achieved. Upper respiratory tract infections are the most common reported adverse events, while more serious infections are rarely encountered in dermatologic conditions. The latter are likely in patients who develop lymphopenia, with higher drug doses and in patients over 65 years of age. A careful watch must be maintained for development of tuberculosis, even if baseline testing was negative and even after prophylaxis has been completed (in case the drug is continued beyond that duration). Development of herpes zoster on treatment, although an uncommon occurrence with dermatologic use, requires treatment interruption until the episode resolves.

The following laboratory monitoring needs to be done on follow-up in patients where prolonged use is planned or expected:

- **Complete blood counts:** CBC monitoring is required at 4–8 weeks of treatment and then 3 monthly thereafter. Any dose increase should also be followed by repeat assessment after 4–6 weeks. Interrupt dosing if hemoglobin falls by >2 g/dL or falls to <8 g/dL. The drug also needs to be stopped if absolute neutrophil count reaches < 500/mm^3 and interruption is required to allow recovery if the same is between 500 and 1,000/mm^3, until it reaches 1,000/mm^3. An absolute lymphocyte count <500/mm^3 predisposes the patient to a higher risk of serious infections and hence requires drug discontinuation. Absolute lymphocyte counts over 750/mm^3 require no dose adjustment, a count of 500–750/mm^3 on two sequential measures suggests a dose reduction or temporary cessation until the count is >750/mm^3 (at which point recommencement can be done).

  Abrocitinib's use has been associated with increased incidence of thrombocytopenia in clinical trials, with maximum effects being observed within 4 weeks, after which the platelet count returned toward baseline despite continued therapy. Adverse outcomes following thrombocytopenia have been reported in six patients who were on 200 mg dose and none with 100 mg dose. Abrocitinib associated reduction in absolute lymphocyte counts also tends to occur in the first 4 weeks of treatment.
- **Liver function testing:** Liver enzyme elevations have been observed with JAKis, especially tofacitinib and baricitinib, and hence, monitoring is required. Though mostly mild and transient, enzyme values above three times the upper limit of normal (ULN) occur in 1–2% of patients on tofacitinib and baricitinib and in <1% of patients on abrocitinib. Severe involvement has however only been described in occasional reports.[20]
- **Lipid profile:** Dyslipidemia is generally seen within 6 weeks of starting the drug; hence, a repeat assessment should be performed at about 4–6 weeks of treatment. The effect of these lipid parameter elevations on cardiovascular morbidity and mortality has not been determined and treatment of any abnormalities detected should be as per existing clinical guidelines for hyperlipidemia management. The elevations do not routinely require treatment discontinuation and changes are reversible on treatment discontinuation.[21]
- **Creatine phosphokinase (CPK):** CPK elevations have been occasionally reported with JAKis, but symptomatic elevations are uncommon and mainly reported with baricitinib.[22,23]
- Consideration should be given to an *annual skin examination* as evidence suggests an increased risk of nonmelanoma skin cancers with tofacitinib, possibly due to prior exposure to methotrexate and tumor necrosis factor (TNF) inhibitors.[5,6]
- **Disease activity** should be monitored regularly to enable stopping of the agents
- The following two **scores are used to predict and suspect pulmonary embolism** and can be used in suspect cases (**Box 2 and Table 1**):

BOX 2 | **PERC criteria.**

- *Age* < 50 years
- Pulse < 100 beats/min
- SaO$_2$ ≥ 95%
- No hemoptysis, estrogen use, surgery/trauma w/ hospitalization in last 4 weeks
- No prior VTE
- No unilateral leg swelling

(PERC: pulmonary embolism rule-out criteria; VTE: venous thromboembolism)
Source: Thromb Haemost. 2008;6:772.

TABLE 1	Wells criteria for PE.	
Criteria		**Points**
PE is the most likely diagnosis or suspected DVT		3 each
HR > 100 beats/min or prior DVT/PE		1.5 each
Immobilization/surgery in last 4 weeks		1.5
Hemoptysis or active malignancy		1 each
If ≤ 4: PE unlikely (7.8% PE rate)		
If > 4: PE likely (40.7% PE rate)		
Clinical probability of PE	**Points**	**Probability of Dz**
Low	<2	3.6%
Medium	2–6	20.5%
High	>6	66.7%

(DVT: deep vein thrombosis; HR: heart rate; PE: pulmonary embolism)

Source: Thromb Haemost. 2000;83:416.

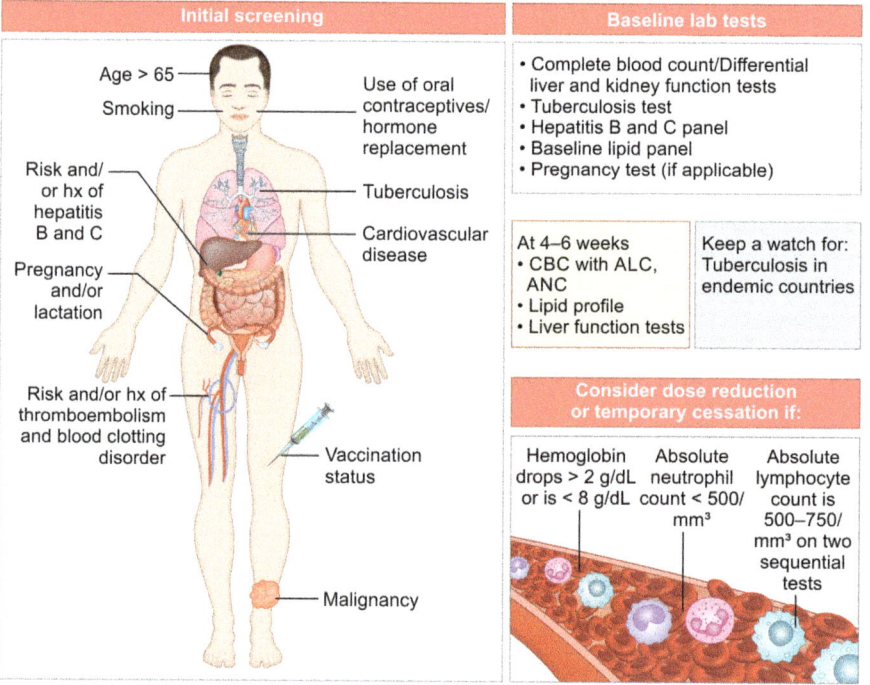

(CBC: complete blood count; ALC: absolute lymphocyte count; ANC: absolute neutrophil count; hx: history)

FIG. 1: Baseline and follow-up assessment for treatment with JAK inhibitors.

An online calculator is also available for the same at: https://www.mdcalc.com/calc/115/wells-criteria-pulmonary-embolism

■ CONCLUSION

An overview of the salient investigations is depicted in **Figure 1**. While the cost may be a constraint, some of adverse effects like dyslipidemia are transient and, in most cases, do not warrant discontinuation. Liver dysfunction is uncommonly seen, mainly with a concomitant liver dysfunction consequent to prior hepatotoxic drug use. IGRA is an expensive test but, TB being a labelled side effect should be investigated for in all cases. Notably in India, some tofacitinib manufacturing companies provide free laboratory tests to patients initiating treatment with tofacitinib, and this can help obviate the costs of initial therapy.

REFERENCES

1. Muddebihal A, Khurana A, Sardana K. JAK inhibitors in dermatology: the road travelled and path ahead, a narrative review. Expert Rev Clin Pharmacol. 2023;16(4):279-95.
2. FDA. Xeljanz/Xeljanz XR. [online] Available from https://www.accessdata.fda.gov/drugsatfda_docs/label/2018/203214s018lbl.pdf [Last accessed January, 2024].
3. FDA. Olumiant. [online] Available from https://www.accessdata.fda.gov/drugsatfda_docs/label/2022/207924s006lbl.pdf [Last accessed January, 2024].
4. Pfizer. Cibinqo$_{TM}$ (abrocitinib). [online] Available from https://cdn.pfizer.com/pfizercom/USPI_Med_Guide_CIBINQO_Abrocitinib_tablet.pdf [Last accessed January, 2024].
5. Nash P, Kerschbaumer A, Dörner T, Dougados M, Fleischmann RM, Geissler K, et al. Points to consider for the treatment of immune-mediated inflammatory diseases with Janus kinase inhibitors: a consensus statement. Ann Rheum Dis. 2021;80(1):71-87.
6. Samuel C, Cornman H, Kambala A, Kwatra SG. A Review on the Safety of Using JAK Inhibitors in Dermatology: Clinical and Laboratory Monitoring. Dermatol Ther (Heidelb). 2023;13(3):729-49.
7. Wang ST, Tseng CW, Hsu CW, Tung CH, Huang KY, Lu MC, et al. Reactivation of hepatitis B virus infection in patients with rheumatoid arthritis receiving tofacitinib. Int J Rheum Dis. 2021;24(11):1362-9.
8. Chen YM, Huang WN, Liao TL, Chen JP, Yang SS, Chen HH, et al. Comparisons of hepatitis C viral replication in patients with rheumatoid arthritis receiving tocilizumab, abatacept and tofacitinib therapy. Ann Rheum Dis. 2019;78(6):849-50.
9. Serling-Boyd N, Mohareb AM, Kim AY, Hyle EP, Wallace ZS. The use of tocilizumab and tofacitinib in patients with resolved hepatitis B infection: a case series. Ann Rheum Dis. 2021;80(2):274-6.
10. Álvaro-Gracia JM, García-Llorente JF, Valderrama M, Gomez S, Montoro M. Update on the Safety Profile of Tofacitinib in Rheumatoid Arthritis from Clinical Trials to Real-World Studies: A Narrative Review. Rheumatol Ther. 2021;8(1):17-40.
11. Winthrop KL, Park SH, Gul A, Cardiel MH, Gomez-Reino JJ, Tanaka Y, et al. Tuberculosis and other opportunistic infections in tofacitinib-treated patients with rheumatoid arthritis. Ann Rheum Dis. 2016;75(6):1133-8.
12. Ytterberg SR, Bhatt DL, Mikuls TR, Koch GG, Fleischmann R, Rivas JL, et al.; ORAL Surveillance Investigators. Cardiovascular and Cancer Risk with Tofacitinib in Rheumatoid Arthritis. N Engl J Med. 2022;386(4):316-26.
13. Ji X, Hu L, Wang Y, Man S, Liu X, Song C, et al. Risk of tuberculosis in patients with rheumatoid arthritis treated with biological and targeted drugs: meta-analysis of randomized clinical trials. Chin Med J (Engl). 2022;135(4):409-15.
14. Cohen SB, Tanaka Y, Mariette X, Curtis JR, Lee EB, Nash P, et al. Long-term safety of tofacitinib up to 9.5 years: a comprehensive integrated analysis of the rheumatoid arthritis clinical development programme. RMD Open. 2020;6(3):e001395.
15. Nash P, Kerschbaumer A, Dörner T, Dougados M, Fleischmann RM, Geissler K, et al. Points to consider for the treatment of immune-mediated inflammatory diseases with Janus kinase inhibitors: a consensus statement. Ann Rheum Dis. 2021;80(1):71-87.
16. Gavegnano C, Brehm JH, Dupuy FP, Talla A, Ribeiro SP, Kulpa DA, et al. Novel mechanisms to inhibit HIV reservoir seeding using Jak inhibitors. PLoS Pathog. 2017;13(12):e1006740.
17. Gavegnano C, Detorio M, Montero C, Bosque A, Planelles V, Schinazi RF. Ruxolitinib and tofacitinib are potent and selective inhibitors of HIV-1 replication and virus reactivation in vitro. Antimicrob Agents Chemother. 2014;58(4):1977-86.
18. Marconi VC, Moser C, Gavegnano C, Deeks SG, Lederman MM, Overton ET, et al. Randomized Trial of Ruxolitinib in Antiretroviral-Treated Adults With Human Immunodeficiency Virus. Clin Infect Dis. 2022;74:95-104.

19. Hoff P, Walther M, Wesselmann H, Weinerth J, Feist E, Ohrndorf S. Erfolgreiche Behandlung eines adulten Morbus Still mit Tofacitinib bei einer HIV-2-positiven Patientin [Successful treatment of adult Still's disease with tofacitinib in a HIV-2 positive female patient]. Z Rheumatol. 2020;79(10):1046-9.
20. Mardani M, Mohammadshahi J, Abolghasemi S, Teimourpour R. Drug-induced liver injury due to tofacitinib: a case report. J Med Case Rep. 2023;17(1):97.
21. Sands BE, Taub PR, Armuzzi A, Friedman GS, Moscariello M, Lawendy N, et al. Tofacitinib Treatment Is Associated With Modest and Reversible Increases in Serum Lipids in Patients With Ulcerative Colitis. Clin Gastroenterol Hepatol. 2020;18(1):123-132.e3.
22. Anjara P, Jiang M, Mundae M. Symptomatic elevation creatine kinase following treatment of rheumatoid arthritis with baricitinib. Clin Rheumatol. 2020;39(2):613-4.
23. Panaccione R, Isaacs JD, Chen LA, Wang W, Marren A, Kwok K, et al. Characterization of Creatine Kinase Levels in Tofacitinib-Treated Patients with Ulcerative Colitis: Results from Clinical Trials. Dig Dis Sci. 2021;66(8):2732-4.3.

CHAPTER 13

Common Janus Kinase Inhibitor Drugs

Kabir Sardana, Sunil Dogra, Shikha Shah

"History is a great teacher"
— George Santayana

Overview	
• Introduction	• Topical Tofacitinib
• Tofacitinib	• Baricitinib

■ INTRODUCTION

While various generations of Janus kinase inhibitor (JAKib) are mentioned in the book (see Chapter 3), India remains a price-sensitive market, and in spite of the varied drugs, tofacitinib still remains the preferred drug. Also it has a long history of usage by rheumatology, and history is the greatest leveler and gives confidence about its usage.

While a precis of the drugs is given in Chapter 3, remember that the **selectivity principles** are based on in vitro whole-blood cytokine assays and plasma pharmacokinetics that assess the JAK-dependent cytokine receptor inhibition profiles of tofacitinib, baricitinib, upadacitinib, and filgotinib, at exposure levels estimated to provide clinically meaningful responses in patients with rheumatoid arthritis (RA). Although in vitro potency differences between JAKibs are apparent, cytokine receptor inhibition profiles across a broad range of pathways are similar after accounting for plasma protein binding, blood-to-plasma ratio, and clinical exposure. There are a few small numerical differences between JAKibs in cytokine receptor inhibition percentages.

Thus **tofacitinib** has a numerically greater relative inhibition of most **JAK1/3**-mediated common γ chain cytokine receptors [interleukin 2 (IL-2), IL-4, IL-7, and IL-15] versus baricitinib, upadacitinib, and filgotinib. Inhibition of **JAK1/JAK2**-mediated cytokine receptors [interferon c (IFN-c) and granulocyte colony-stimulating factor (G-CSF)] and JAK2-mediated cytokine receptors (thrombopoietin, IL-3, and GM-CSF) are greater with **upadacitinib** versus other JAKibs.[1] These minor differences in predicted cytokine receptor inhibition between JAKibs suggested that there is limited differences between their clinical profiles in RA and thus may not be clinically relevant. Due to market availability in India we are discussing tofacitinib and baricitinib while a summary of the other drugs is detailed in chapter.

■ TOFACITINIB

Tofacitinib has been evaluated for its inhibitory effect against JAKs, and it inhibits JAK3 at an IC50 of 55 nM and JAK1 and JAK2 with IC50 values of 15.1 nM and 77.4 nM, respectively. Thus, tofacitinib is a JAK1 and 3 > JAK2 inhibitor.

It is available in both oral and topical formulation. Here, it is notable that there are a few manufacturers of the drug and the quality is largely comparable. The belief that the generics are in any ways inferior to the originator brand is a misplaced concept. We have used both and do not find any marked variations in efficacy.

Dose

Orally, it is available as 5 mg tablet, 11 mg extended release (XR) tablet, and 1 mg/mL oral suspension.

For children (2-17 years) the dose is:
- *40 kg*: 5 mg BD
- *20-40 kg*: 4 mg BD
- *10-20 kg*: 3.2 mg twice daily

Renal (severe) and moderate hepatic impairment: 5 mg OD when indicated dose is 5 mg BID; 5 mg BID when the indicated dose is 10 mg BID.

In **clinical practice,** start the drug at 5 mg OD and titrate depending on patient response. Maintenance with low dose 5 mg OD or 5 mg alternate day is necessary due to high relapse rates. We have used the drug up to 6 years continuously with no adverse effects.

Pharmacokinetics

After oral administration peak plasma levels are achieved in 30 minutes. Bioavailability of the drug is 74%, while 40% of the drug is bound to plasma proteins.

Half-life: 3 hours—the drug undergoes hepatic (70%) and renal (30%) excretion.

Pharmacodynamics

Pharmacodynamic effects: Treatment with tofacitinib for up to 6 months in RA patients was linked to dose-dependent reduction in circulating CD16/56+ natural killer (NK) cells, with greatest reduction thought to occur 8–10 weeks after starting treatment. After discontinuation of treatment, the depressed lymphocyte population reverted to normal basal state in 2–6 weeks.

Food and Drug Administration-approved Indications

It is currently United States Food and Drug Administration (US FDA) approved for moderate to severe active RA, psoriatic arthritis (PsA) (5 mg BD and 11 mg XR) [US and European Medicines Agency (EMA)], ulcerative colitis, juvenile idiopathic arthritis, ankylosing spondylitis, and alopecia areata (AA).

Off label is used for varied indications (**Box 1**). Also see Chapter 10.
- **Alopecia areata:** The existing evidence indicates that the dose ranges from **5 to 15 mg** though there are poor/nonresponders. The hair regrowth generally begins after 6–8 weeks of treatment and full regrowth can be expected between 3 and 14 months in responders. Better clinical outcomes have been linked to shorter disease duration and peribulbar inflammation on pretreatment scalp biopsies, while patients with disease duration >10 years are less likely to respond to tofacitinib. The likelihood of

> **BOX 1** **Off label uses of tofacitinib.**
>
> - *Connective tissue disorders*: Dermatomyositis, systemic sclerosis, morphea, and recalcitrant lupus erythematosus
> - *Immunobullous diseases*: Bullous pemphigoid and pemphigus
> - *Dermatitis*: Refractory eczemas, hand eczema, parthenium dermatitis, chronic actinic dermatitis, and atopic dermatitis
> - *Granulomatous disorders*: Granuloma annulare, necrobiosis lipoidica, and sarcoidosis
> - *Lichenoid disorders*: Lichen planus (LP), lichen planopilaris, and hypertrophic LP
> - *Others*: Palmoplantar pustulosis, cutaneous polyarteritis nodosa, prurigo nodularis, vitiligo, Behçet's disease, and amyloidosis

complete regrowth decreases with each year leading to 10 years of complete scalp hair loss. Patients with AA show better response compared to patients with alopecia totalis/alopecia universalis (AT/AU), although the latter can also show a remarkable response to treatment.[2] Unfortunately, relapse is seen in around 25% patients a median of 8.5 weeks after cessation of treatment, necessitating prolonged maintenance.[3]

Notably the drug has been shown to be *better than* existing immunosuppressive agents (ISAs) and is useful even as monotherapy. According to a recent study, out of 74 patients (18 treated with tofacitinib, 26 treated with conventional oral treatment (steroid/cyclosporine), and 30 treated with diphenylcyclopropenone, after 6 months, 44.4% of patients in the tofacitinib group, 37.5% in the conventional oral treatment group, and 11.1% in the diphenylcyclopropenone group had improved their Severity of Alopecia Tool (SALT) score by 50%. Adverse reactions were seen in 10% of patients in the tofacitinib group, 73.1% in the conventional oral treatment group, and 10% in the diphenylcyclopropenone group during the treatment. After 6 months of treatment, oral tofacitinib was better than diphenylcyclopropenone immunotherapy and more tolerated than traditional oral therapy.[4]

- **Psoriatic arthritis**: Tofacitinib has been approved by various drug regulatory agencies as well as Indian drug regulatory agency Central Drugs Standard Control Organization (CDSCO) for use in PsA in the dose of 5 mg twice daily.
- **Psoriasis**: Tofacitinib has been extensively studied in psoriasis. A pooled analysis was carried out by Strober BE et al. comprising 5,204 patient-years of tofacitinib treatment and concluded that tofacitinib **10 mg BID** showed greater efficacy than 5 mg BID.[5] However, the efficacy was lower in patients with baseline Psoriasis Area and Severity Index (PASI) < 20, prior systemic therapy and bodyweight > 90 kg at baseline. A meta-analysis conducted by Pfizer reported that the efficacy of tofacitinib 5 mg BD was similar to that of oral methotrexate 15 mg and etanercept 25 mg twice weekly, and higher than that of acitretin and apremilast, while the efficacy of tofacitinib 10 mg BID was comparable to that of injectable tumor necrosis factor (TNF) antagonists and cyclosporine, and greater than apremilast, acitretin, methotrexate, and fumarates.[6] In our experience the drug is not markedly effective in psoriasis vulgaris (see Chapter 6).
- **Atopic dermatitis (AD):** Although the drug has not been evaluated in large trials, clinical use demonstrates good efficacy. Tofacitinib 5 mg once/twice daily for 14 days was found to be to efficacious in six patients with moderate-to-severe refractory AD who had failed conventional treatment, and resulted in a 55% decrease in Severity Scoring of Atopic Dermatitis (SCORAD) with no adverse effects. (Also refer to Chapters 5 and 8).
- **Vitiligo:** Tofacitinib has also been shown to induce repigmentation of vitiligo (mainly on face and other sun exposed sites) in case reports/series and small studies, in oral as well as topical forms. (Refer to Chapter 7).

Adverse Effects

While the side effects have been detailed in Chapter 11, there is a large data which analyzed continuous use of tofacitinib spanning **9.5** years of cumulative exposure in >7,000 patients, a good safety profile was established. The only issue is thromboembolic events which are seen only in special populations, malignancies [nonmelanoma skin cancer (NMSC)], and herpes zoster (nonserious and serious). Thus the drug is safe and the side effects reported in RA literature are due to the concomitant use of oral steroids and also the fact that RA can predispose to certain side effects. In India TB is a risk and thus a baseline evaluation (Mantoux/IGRA) is a must. The most common side effect remains dyslipidemia and is generally not a serious issue. Apart from flare of tinea corporis, we have not noted any markedly different adverse effects, in the last 4 years of use in RML hospital.

Tofacitinib is primarily metabolized by CYP3A4. The total daily dose should be halved in patients receiving potent CYP3A4 inhibitors, and in patients receiving concomitant medicinal products resulting in both moderate inhibition of CYP3A4 and potent inhibition of CYP2C19 (e.g., fluconazole).

■ TOPICAL TOFACITINIB

It is available as 1% and 2% ointment and gels. While the industry claims it be effective, we have not found it to mirror the exuberant support it receives from sponsored sessions and without adjuvant drugs the results do not justify the high cost of the preparation.

Conclusion

This drug has been cost-effective and is superior to oral glucocorticosteroids and a host of ISAs due to its ability to inhibit multiple cytokines and Th-cell lines without affecting bystander cells. It has the potential to treat a host of Th1- and Th2-mediated disorders and it would likely replace oral GCS in many indications in the near future.

■ REFERENCES

1. Traves PG, Murray B, Campigotto F, Galien R, Meng A, Di Paolo JA, et al. JAK selectivity and the implications for clinical inhibition of pharmacodynamic cytokine signalling by filgotinib, upadacitinib, tofacitinib and baricitinib. Ann Rheum Dis. 2021;80:865-75.
2. Jabbari A, Sansaricq F, Cerise J, Chen JC, Bitterman A, Ulerio G, et al. An Open-Label Pilot Study to Evaluate the Efficacy of Tofacitinib in Moderate to Severe Patch-type Alopecia Areata, Totalis, and Universalis. J Invest Dermatol. 2018;138(7):1539-45.
3. Hogan S, Wang S, Ibrahim O, Piliang M, Bergfeld W. Long-Term Treatment with Tofacitinib in Severe Alopecia Areata: An Update. J Clin Aesthet Dermatol. 2019;12(6):12-4.
4. Shin JW, Huh CH, Kim MW, Lee JS, Kwon O, Cho S, et al. Comparison of the Treatment Outcome of Oral Tofacitinib with Other Conventional Therapies in Refractory Alopecia Totalis and Universalis: A Retrospective Study. Acta Derm Venereol. 2019;99(1):41-6.
5. Papp KA, Menter MA, Abe M, Elewski B, Feldman SR, Gottlieb AB, et al. Tofacitinib, an oral Janus kinase inhibitor, for the treatment of chronic plaque psoriasis: results from two randomized, placebo-controlled, phase III trials. Br J Dermatol. 2015;173(4):949-61.
6. Strober BE, Gottlieb AB, van de Kerkhof PCM, Puig L, Bachelez H, Chouela E, et al. Benefit-risk profile of tofacitinib in patients with moderate-to-severe chronic plaque psoriasis: pooled analysis across six clinical trials. Br J Dermatol. 2019;180(1):67-75.

BARICITINIB

Introduction

Baricitinib belongs to the class of "oral small molecule". It acts by competitive inhibition of "Janus kinase (JAK) family", primarily targeting JAK1 and JAK2 subtypes. Initially approved for RA, baricitinib is now US FDA approved for the management in dermatology in the management of conditions such as AD and AA. Dermatologists are encouraged to acquire comprehensive knowledge regarding this emerging oral small molecule in order to enhance its application across various dermatoses along with carefully monitoring for potential adverse events.

Mechanism of Action

The JAK family is part of a subset of "nonreceptor protein tyrosine kinases", and it is associated with intracellular domains of various types of cytokine receptors. When certain cytokines bind to their respective receptors, JAKs become activated, initiating downstream signaling pathways. Depending on the cytokines present, these kinases can form homo- or heterodimers, leading to autophosphorylation. Subsequently, this autophosphorylation process phosphorylates and recruits "STAT proteins" (signal transducer and activator of transcription protein). Ultimately, this cascade of events results in the transcription of various types of inflammatory mediators.[1]

Baricitinib is a preferential inhibitor of JAK1/2. It interferes with JAK, thereby preventing its autophosphorylation. This further prevents its attachment to STAT proteins. STAT proteins, when unphosphorylated, lack the capacity to trigger downstream transcription of different types of proinflammatory mediators. Through its selective binding to JAK1/2, it also exerts anti-inflammatory as well as antiviral responses, particularly by modulation of IFN-alpha, IFN-beta, and IFN-gamma downstream signaling pathways.[2]

Efficacy and Uses

Baricitinib has been used across various indications in dermatology, both on and off the label with encouraging results. The approved uses of baricitinib in dermatology have been summarized in **Table 1**.

Apart from dermatology indications, baricitinib is already US FDA approved for treatment of RA in June 2018 and coronavirus disease 2019 (COVID-19) in May 2022. Baricitinib is the first and was the only systemic drug to be approved in AA, but recently ritlecitinib has been approved for AA. In a recent systematic review of baricitinib in AA, it was seen that significant proportion of AA patients achieve SALT score of ≤ 20 when compared with placebo with no serious side effects.[10] It was seen in a recent study that patients may be switched between tofacitinib and baricitinib with maintenance of response; a few patients on partial recovery with tofacitinib showed complete regrowth on baricitinib (**Figs. 1A to D**).[11]

In India, the CDSCO initially had granted "emergency use authorization" for the use of baricitinib (in combination with remdesivir) in COVID-19 cases. However, the Indian Council of Medical Research (ICMR) later withdrew this authorization due to inconclusive evidence regarding its efficacy. Despite this, generic versions of baricitinib have been introduced in the Indian market without patent waivers. Regarding approval, there is an ongoing process to obtain permission for its use in RA, and trials are currently underway to explore its potential application in dermatological indications. Comprehensive data from robust Indian studies are still pending.

TABLE 1	Baricitinib in dermatology: Approved indications, dosing, and efficacy reported in key clinical trials.				
Disease	Mechanism	Approval	Indication	Dose	Efficacy
Alopecia areata (AA)[3]	Blocks IFN-γ signaling, decreasing IL-15 production and cytotoxic T-cells[4]	US FDA, June 2022	Severe AA (defined as "50% or greater scalp hair loss")	• 2 mg once daily, increase to 4 mg if inadequate response • *Alopecia subtotalis/ totalis*: Can start with 4 mg/day	*BRAVE-AA1* and *BRAVE-AA2* trials:[5,6] Regrowth in the hair was found to be significantly superior to placebo at 36 weeks
Atopic dermatitis (AD)[7]	Inhibits Th2 cytokines like IL-4, IL-5, IL-13, IL-22, IL-31, and TSLP, upregulates filaggrin[8]	EMA, September 2020	Moderate to severe AD in age > 18 years	4 mg once daily	*BREEZE AD* trials[9]: Improvement in patient and physician reported outcomes over 16 weeks with sustained longer term efficacy studied up to 68 weeks

(EMA: European Medicines Agency; IFN-γ: interferon gamma; IL: interleukin; TSLP: thymic stromal lymphopoietin)

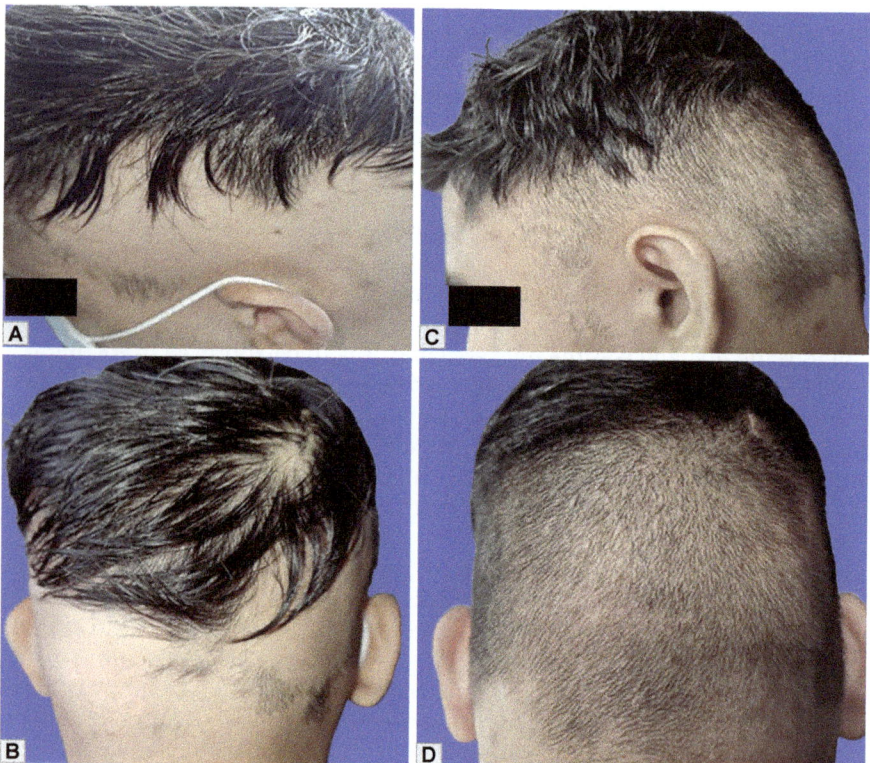

FIGS. 1A TO D: (A and B) A 23-year-old male with alopecia areata showed relapse of ophiasis while on tofacitinib 5 mg twice daily for 6 months. The patient was switched to baricitinib 4 mg/day. (C and D) After 12 weeks of therapy, there was regrowth with no disease progression.

Off-label Uses

Baricitinib has been tried off-label across various other dermatoses.[2,12,13]
- *Papulosquamous/lichenoid and eczematous*: Psoriasis, lichen planus, and prurigo
- *Connective tissue diseases/sclerosing disorders*: Lupus erythematosus, systemic sclerosis, dermatomyositis, chronic graft-versus-host disease, lichen sclerosus
- *Cicatricial alopecias*: Folliculitis decalvans, lichen planopilaris, and frontal fibrosing alopecia
- *Neutrophilic/granulomatous disorders*: Pyoderma gangrenosum, Sweet's syndrome, and granuloma annulare
- *Miscellaneous*: Vitiligo, pemphigoid disorders, interferonopathies, and other autoinflammatory disorders such as CANDLE and VEXAS syndromes, livedoid vasculopathy, progressive nodular histiocytosis, genodermatoses like Darier disease, Hutchinson-Gilford progeria, and epidermolysis bullosa pruriginosa.

Side Effects and Special Considerations

The various adverse effects of baricitinib have been summarized in **Table 2** and the Indian experience with the drug is yet not extensive to validate the side effects reported in western literature.[14]

Similar to all JAKibs, baricitinib has boxed warnings and precautions, summarized in **Table 3**.[14]

Baricitinib should be avoided in pregnancy, lactation, and severe renal or hepatic impairment, while the use in pediatric and geriatric population is to be on a case-to-case basis. It should not be used in conjunction with other JAKibs or disease-modifying antirheumatic drugs (DMARDs).

TABLE 2	Adverse effects of baricitinib.
Frequency	**Adverse effects**
Common (≥1% patients on baricitinib for dermatological indications)	• Nausea, fatigue, abdominal pain, weight gain, and headache • Acne and folliculitis • *Infections*: Upper and lower respiratory tract infections, genital candidiasis, herpes zoster, and urinary tract infections • *Laboratory abnormalities*: Hyperlipidemia, elevated blood creatine phosphokinase, liver enzyme elevations, anemia, and neutropenia
Rare, serious (<1% cases)	Arterial thrombosis, fungal skin infections lymphopenia, and B-cell lymphoma
Delayed (seen >52 weeks or in postmarketing surveillance)	Deep vein thrombosis and pulmonary embolism, drug hypersensitivity (urticaria, angioedema, and rash), and nonmelanoma skin cancer

TABLE 3	Boxed warnings and precautions with baricitinib.
Boxed warnings	**Warnings/Precautions**
• Infections • Malignancies • Thrombosis • Major adverse cardiovascular events	• Hypersensitivity • Gastrointestinal perforation • Laboratory abnormalities • Vaccinations

Baricitinib does not affect the cytochrome P450 enzymes significantly. Baricitinib is a substrate for OAT3 (organic anionic transporter 3). Hence, the dose of baricitinib needs to be halved with concurrent use of strong OAT3 inhibitors like probenecid.[14]

Limited studies have been conducted where in baricitinib has been used specifically for dermatological purposes. Hence, the data from its use in rheumatology cannot be extrapolated, because RA pathogenesis has a background risk of infections and cardiovascular risk.[15] Therefore, existing literature needs to be critically assessed, and attention should be given to forthcoming practice-based literature in various settings.

While the "labeled warnings" are currently in place, caution is particularly important in specific subgroups:[16]
- Aged over 50 or under 18 years (due to the risks associated with age and the lack of safety data in long-term)
- Elevated baseline risk of having a possible malignancy (personal or family history related to malignancies and history of smoking)
- Patients already having the presence of ≥1 cardiovascular risk factors (such as diabetes, hyperlipidemia, and hypertension).

Monitoring

The investigations required for baricitinib initiation and monitoring while on treatment has been summarized in **Table 4**.[17]

TABLE 4	Clinical and laboratory monitoring while on baricitinib.	
Baseline evaluation		
• Thorough history and examination focusing on any infections, comorbidities, and malignancies/lymphoproliferative conditions • *Screening for infections*: Hepatitis B and C • Screening for latent/active tuberculosis • Immunization against herpes zoster and streptococcal pneumonia; live and attenuated viral vaccines to be avoided on therapy • Hemogram, liver function tests, renal function tests, and fasting lipid profile		
Follow-up evaluation and monitoring		
Laboratory parameter	Possible adverse events	Monitoring
Complete blood counts	• Neutropenia • Lymphopenia • Anemia • Thrombocythemia	• Baseline, every 4–8 weeks after initiation followed by 3 monthly • *Stop*: Absolute lymphocyte count (ALC) < 500 cells/μL, absolute neutrophil count (ANC) < 1,000 cells/μL, or hemoglobin level < 8 g/dL
Liver function tests	Liver enzyme elevations	• Baseline, every 4 weeks till first 12 weeks, followed by 3 monthly • *Stop*: If drug-induced liver injury is suspected with >5 times elevations of AST or ALT from upper normal limit (UNL)
Lipid profile	• Hypercholesterolemia • Hypertriglyceridemia • Increase in LDL and HDL levels	• Baseline, at 12 weeks • Treat the hyperlipidemia as per guidelines

(ALT: alanine transaminase; AST: aspartate transaminase; HDL: high-density lipoprotein; LDL: low-density lipoprotein)

Summary and Expert Opinion

Baricitinib has its place in management of subset of patients with severe AA and AD where other therapies have failed. There is reasonable efficacy and safety in literature for its use; however, clinicians should be wary for its potential serious adverse events. Data reporting is crucial to generate more evidence regarding its safety in dermatological conditions rather than relying on data from rheumatology. The horizon of JAKibs including baricitinib is expanding, and the drug has been under exploration for a plethora of "immune"-mediated diseases where careful downstream regulation of transcription factors can prove a game changer, especially in refractory cases. Baricitinib is being placed in the management of systemic lupus erythematosus with good evidence in recent times. Its role is also being studied in hidradenitis suppurativa and psoriasis with impetus.[18,19]

The evolution of JAKibs has certainly proven fortuitous in autoimmune conditions that may be recalcitrant to many other conventional modalities. The results of baricitinib are most encouraging in AA and AD, but the scope does not end there as it targets a wide array of downstream mediators. There are certain limitations as well, including uncertainty of response, lack of safety data in dermatological settings, and especially in the pediatric population where AA and AD, the two important indications of baricitinib, are usually encountered.[20] Nevertheless, baricitinib and other future selective JAKibs do possess the potential to alter the "therapeutic paradigm" of several inflammatory dermatoses, making it important for dermatologists to be well versed with its nuances.

■ REFERENCES

1. Damsky W, King BA. JAK inhibitors in dermatology: the promise of a new drug class. J Am Acad Dermatol. 2017;76:736-44.
2. Dogra S, Shah S, Sharma A, Chhabra S, Narang T. Emerging Role of Baricitinib in Dermatology Practice: All We Need to Know! Indian Dermatol Online J. 2023;14:153-62.
3. Ali E, Owais R, Sheikh A, Shaikh A. Olumniant (Baricitinib) oral tablets: An insight into FDA-approved systemic treatment for Alopecia Areata. Ann Med Surg. 2022;80:104157.
4. Zhang J, Qi F, Dong J, Tan Y, Gao L, Liu F. Application of baricitinib in dermatology. J Inflamm Res. 2022;15:1935.
5. King B, Ko J, Forman S, Ohyama M, Mesinkovska N, Yu G, et al. Efficacy and safety of the oral Janus kinase inhibitor baricitinib in the treatment of adults with alopecia areata: Phase 2 results from a randomized controlled study. J Am Acad Dermatol. 2021;85:847-53.
6. King B, Ohyama M, Kwon O, Zlotogorski A, Ko J, Mesinkovska NA, et al. Two phase 3 trials of Baricitinib for alopecia areata. N Engl J Med. 2022;386:1687-99.
7. Radi G, Simonetti O, Rizzetto G, Diotallevi F, Molinelli E, Offidani A. Baricitinib: the first jak inhibitor approved in Europe for the treatment of moderate to severe atopic dermatitis in adult patients. Healthcare. 2021;9:1575.
8. Hoy SM. Baricitinib: A Review in Moderate to Severe Atopic Dermatitis. Am J Clin Dermatol. 2022:1-2.
9. Silverberg JI, Simpson EL, Wollenberg A, Bissonnette R, Kabashima K, DeLozier AM, et al. Long-term efficacy of baricitinib in adults with moderate to severe atopic dermatitis who were treatment responders or partial responders: an extension study of 2 randomized clinical trials. JAMA Dermatol. 2021;157:691-9.
10. Mahmoud AM. Effectiveness and safety of baricitinib in patients with alopecia areata: a systematic review and Meta-analysis of randomized controlled trials. Curr Med Res Opin. 2023;39:249-57.
11. Kazmi A, Moussa A, Bokhari L, Bhoyrul B, Joseph S, Chitreddy V, et al. Switching between tofacitinib and baricitinib in alopecia areata: A review of clinical response. J Am Acad Dermatol. 2023;89:1248-50.
12. Corbella-Bagot L, Riquelme-McLoughlin C, Morgado-Carrasco D. Long-Term Safety Profile and Off-Label Use of JAK Inhibitors in Dermatological Disorders. Actas Dermosifiliogr. 2023;114:784-801.

13. Shah A, Yumeen S, Qureshi A, Saliba E. Off-Label Use of Baricitinib in Dermatology. J Drugs Dermatol. 2023;22:795-801.
14. Olumiant (Baricitinib). (2022). U.S. Food and Drug Administration. [online] Available from https://www.accessdata.fda.gov/drugsatfda_docs/label/2022/207924s006lbl.pdf [Last accessed March, 2024].
15. Hoisnard L, Lebrun-Vignes B, Maury S, Mahevas M, El Karoui K, Roy L, et al. Adverse events associated with JAK inhibitors in 126,815 reports from the WHO pharmacovigilance database. Sci Rep. 2022;12(1):7140.
16. Murphrey M, Waldman RA, Durso T, Grant-Kels JM. Special editorial: When prescribing Janus kinase inhibitors for dermatologic conditions, be mindful of the Food and Drug Administration's September 1, 2021, data safety communication. J Am Acad Dermatol. 2022;86:42-3.
17. Ahmad A, Zaheer M, Balis FJ. Baricitinib. StatPearls [Internet]. Treasure Island (FL): StatPearls Publishing; 2021.
18. Maronese CA, Moltrasio C, Genovese G, Marzano AV. Biologics for Hidradenitis suppurativa: evolution of the treatment paradigm. Expert Rev Clin Immunol. 2023:1-21.
19. Funk PJ, Perche PO, Singh R, Kelly KA, Feldman SR. Comparing available JAK inhibitors for treating patients with psoriasis. Expert Rev Clin Immunol. 2022;18:281-94.
20. Muddebihal A, Khurana A, Sardana K. JAK inhibitors in dermatology: the road travelled and path ahead, a narrative review. Expert Rev Clin Pharmacol. 2023;16:279-95.

Index

Page numbers followed by *b* refer to box, *f* refer to figure, *fc* refer to flowchart, and *t* refer to table.

A

Abrocitinib 29, 30, 37, 40, 42, 58, 61, 62, 66, 84, 87, 88, 92, 99, 104, 112, 115, 121, 129
Absolute lymphocyte count 130
Absolute neutrophil count 130, 140
Acne 66, 77, 115, 122, 139
Activated T cells, nuclear factor of 20
Activin receptor-like kinase inhibitor 52
Acute myeloid leukemia 26
Adalimumab 70, 71*f*, 72*f*
Adenosine triphosphate 31
Alanine transaminase 140
Allergens 56
Allergic contact dermatitis 87, 97
Alopecia areata 19, 29, 30, 39, 43, 46, 47*f*, 48, 49, 51*f*, 78, 98, 111, 112, 134, 138, 138*f*
  immune-pathogenesis of 47*f*
  pathogenesis of 46
  severe 41
  treatment of 49*fc*
Alopecia tool
  score, severity of 48
  severity of 49
Alopecia totalis 46, 51*f*
Alopecia universalis 46
Amphiregulin 14
Amyloidosis 98, 135
Anemia 36, 61, 113, 115, 139, 140
Angioedema 139
Ankylosing spondylitis 32, 39, 41, 42, 112, 134
Ankylosing spondyloarthritis 29
Antibody antagonists 26
Antibody-dependent cell-mediated cytotoxicity 12
Antidepressants 104
Antigen-presenting cell 9, 47, 87
Antihepatitis C antibodies 127
Anti-interleukin-1 beta 19
Antineutrophil cytoplasmic antibody 107
Antiretroviral therapy 128
Anti-tumor necrosis factor 19, 70
Aortic valve sclerosis 117
Appendectomy 121
Apremilast 71
Arterial thrombosis 139
Artery disease, coronary 99
Arthritis 72*f*
  juvenile 29
    idiopathic 41, 61, 134
Aspartate transaminase 140
Asthma 22
Atopic dermatitis 22, 29, 30, 36, 41-43, 55, 56*f*, 57-62, 63*f*, 65, 66, 82, 83, 85*f*, 90-92, 97, 98, 111, 112, 122, 135, 138
  acute phase of 60
  mild-to-moderate 57
  moderate to severe 42, 58
  pathogenesis of 56, 58*t*
  severity scoring of 135
Autoimmune disease 16, 19
Autoimmune disorder 19, 96, 109
  abdominal 73
Autoinflammatory disorders 19, 139
Autoinflammatory syndromes 19
Axial spondyloarthritis 42
Azathioprine 50, 62

B

B cells 3, 34, 106, 107
  activating factor 105
  lymphoma 139
  sensors of 2
B lymphocytes 19
Bacillus Calmette–Guérin vaccination 127
Baricitinib 29, 30, 36, 37, 39, 41, 50, 52, 58, 61, 62, 63*f*, 64, 66, 76, 84, 85*f*, 86-88, 92, 99, 102, 104, 111, 112, 115, 119, 121, 122, 133, 137, 138*f*, 138*t*, 139, 139*b*, 140, 140*t*, 141
  adverse effects of 139*b*

Barzolvolimab 104
Basophils 1
Behçet's disease 135
Bimekizumab 70
Biological disease-modifying antirheumatic drugs 31, 118
Blood creatinine phosphokinase 115
Body mass index 125
Body surface area 76, 77
Brepocitinib 36, 37, 41, 43, 52, 58, 60, 70, 76, 78, 117
Bruton tyrosine kinase 32
Bullous dermatosis 99
Bullous pemphigoid 92, 98, 135

C

Calcineurin inhibitor, topical 49
Candida albicans 13
CANDLE syndromes 139
Cardiac death, sudden 117
Cardiac disease 125
Cardiotrophin 24
Cardiovascular death 117
Cardiovascular system 115, 121
Cells 14
Cellulitis 119
Central nervous system, primary 107
Cerdulatinib 36, 76
Cerebrovascular accident 117
Certolizumab 70
Chemokine 15, 75*f*
  role of 15
Chest X-ray 127
Cholecystectomy 121
Chronic actinic dermatitis 87, 88, 135
Churg–Strauss syndrome 108
Cicatricial alopecias 139
Ciclosporin 62
Ciliary neurotrophic growth factor 24
Colon polyp 121
Colony-stimulating factor 1 receptor 26
Combination therapy 27
Complete blood count 121, 129, 130
Compositae airborne dermatitis 88
Connective tissue diseases 139
Contact dermatitis 115
Coronavirus disease 2019 (COVID-19) 29, 117, 137
  infection 41
Corticosteroid, topical 57, 101

Creatinine phosphokinase 115, 121, 129
Crisaborole 57
Crohn's disease 32, 40, 101
Cryoglobulinemic vasculitis 107
Cyclooxygenase 115
Cyclosporine 49, 50, 51*f*, 62, 85*f*
Cytokine 7*f*, 12-14, 17, 20, 24, 27, 47*f*, 91*f*, 102*f*, 107, 113
  antibodies 26
  balance 11
  experimental inhibitions of 26
  Janus kinase interaction 97*f*
  ligands 37
  mediated pathway 69*f*
  overview of 113*t*
  patterns 12*f*
  receptor 4-6, 37
    classes of 4
  role of 10, 83
  signaling pathway 19, 24
Cytomegalovirus 17
Cytopenia 66*t*
Cytoplasmic tyrosine kinases 74

D

Damage-associated molecular pattern receptors 2
Dapsone 101*f*
Darier disease 139
Decernotinib 37, 41
Deep vein thrombosis 118, 130, 139
Delgocitinib 29, 30, 36, 42, 43, 52, 60, 76, 86, 92, 99, 115, 122
Dendritic cell 1, 4*f*, 34, 56, 69, 103
Dermatitis 135
  herpetiformis 98
Dermatology 30, 138*t*
Dermatomyositis 98, 135, 139
Deucravacitinib 29, 30, 37, 41, 42, 52, 58, 70, 100, 115, 122
Diabetes mellitus 70, 118, 140
Diarrhea 40
Diphenylcyclopropenone 49, 135
Discoid eczema 98
Discoid lupus erythematosus 42, 43
Disease-modifying antirheumatic drugs 139
Diverticulitis 121
Dizziness 115
Dorsal root ganglion 103
Double-blind vehicle control trial 77

Drug
   hypersensitivity 139
   interactions 126
Dual-target Janus kinase inhibitor 51
Dupilumab 63, 64, 84, 86, 92, 104
Dyslipidemia 61, 66, 78, 115, 129

E

Eczema 97, 98
   area and severity index 65, 85, 88
      score 42, 60
   herpeticum 84, 117
Eczematous disorders 82
Elevated blood creatine phosphokinase 139
Elevated creatinine 115
   kinase 115
Elevated lipid parameters 115
Endothelial-mesenchymal transition 105
Eosinophils 1, 83, 103
Epidermal cells 74
Epidermolysis bullosa pruriginosa 98t, 139
Epithelial lining 3
Erythema 76
   multiforme 98
   nodosum leprosum 17
Erythroderma, history of 85f
Erythropoiesis 30
Erythropoietin 4, 20, 24, 35, 112-114
Etanercept 70
Extracellular signal-regulated kinase
   pathways 33

F

Fas ligand 7, 100
Fasting lipid profile 140
Fatigue 139
Fedratinib 29t, 37, 42
Fibrosis, cutaneous 105
Filaggrin mutations 56
Filgotinib 29t, 37t, 40, 42t
Fluconazole 62t, 136
Fluvoxamine 62t
Folliculitis 139
   decalvans 139
Frontal fibrosing alopecia 139
Fungal infectious disorders 119
Fungal skin infections 139
Fusion proteins 26

G

Gastric ulcer 121
Gastroenteritis 121
Gastrointestinal adverse events 119, 120
Gastrointestinal perforation 39, 139
Gastrointestinal tract 101
Genital candidiasis 139t
Genodermatoses 139
Genome-wide association studies 47, 106
Giant cell arteritis 107
Glucocorticoids 99, 106, 125
Glucocorticosteroids, systemic 49
Graft-versus-host disease 29, 43, 112
   chronic 38, 41, 139
   cutaneous 43
Granulocyte-macrophage colony-stimulating
   factor 4, 8, 11, 14, 35, 37, 56, 58, 83, 97,
   112-114, 133
Granulocytes 1
Granuloma annulare 98, 101, 102, 135, 139
Granulomatosis 108
Granulomatous disorders 135, 139
Growth hormone 20, 24, 35, 112, 114
Gusacitinib 36, 61, 99
Guselkumab 70

H

Hair follicles 46
Hand eczema 30, 97, 135
   chronic 42, 43, 88, 97-99, 99t
Headache 44, 66, 77, 115, 121, 139
Heart
   disease, coronary 118
   rate 130
Helminth infestations, cutaneous 92b
Hematological cytopenia 78
Hematopoietic cells 34
Hemogram 140
Hemophagocytic lymphohistiocytosis 101
Henoch–Schönlein purpura 107
Hepatic aminotransferase 115
Hepatic disease, severe 126
Hepatic dysfunction 125
Hepatitis
   B 140
      infection 125, 128
      surface antigen 127
   virus 39, 52

C 140
   infection 125, 128
   virus 52
   profile 127
Hepatocellular carcinoma 26
Herpes simplex 66
   virus infections 17
Herpes viral infections 119
Herpes zoster 39, 61, 64, 66, 113, 115, 136, 139
Hidradenitis suppurativa 42, 43, 98-100
Human immunodeficiency virus 17, 52, 127
   infection 128
Human leukocyte antigen 16, 19
Hutchinson-Gilford progeria 139
Hypercholesterolemia 115, 140
Hypereosinophilic syndrome 26, 98
Hyperkeratosis 103
Hyperlipidemia 113, 115, 139, 140
   management 129
Hyperplasia, delayed-type 103
Hypersensitivity 139
   delayed-type 12
Hypertension 140
   history of 118
Hypertriglyceridemia 140

I

Ifidancitinib 43t, 76t, 78
Immune
   cells 34, 47f
   complex-mediated vasculitis 107
   dysfunction 74t
   regulation 15
   response, activation of 3
   suppression 113
   system 19
Immunity
   adaptive 2f, 19, 74
   cell-mediated 3, 6
   humoral 3
   innate 2f, 74
   mucosal 12
Immunobullous diseases 135
Immunoglobulin 113
   A 99
   E 6, 56, 59, 83
Immunologic memory 3
Immunology 1
Immunosuppressive agent 1, 126

Infections 115, 119, 139
   opportunistic 39, 61
Inflammatory bowel disease 31, 126
Inflammatory disorders 96
Infliximab 70
Influenza 119
Innate lymphoid cells 2, 11, 14, 14f
   five groups of 14
Insect bite reactions 92
Interferon 5, 24, 25, 28, 33, 35, 37, 44, 47, 56, 97, 74, 75, 102, 113, 115
   alpha 68
   gamma 7, 8, 11-15, 34, 47, 56, 83, 100, 112, 138
   release assays 127
Interleukin 5-8, 12-15, 17, 22, 24, 25, 28, 32, 34, 35, 37, 44, 47, 56, 59, 69, 70, 73-75, 83, 91, 97, 99, 103, 104, 112-115, 138
   receptor 58
   transduction signals 24t
Interstitial lung disease 106
Intracellular signal transduction 111
Intralesional steroid injections 48
Irritable bowel syndrome 121
Isoniazid 127
Itacitinib 37t
Itch 90, 93, 98
   relief 91, 92
   scratch 86
   sensation of 91f
Ixekizumab 70b

J

Janus kinase 5, 20, 22, 25, 27-29, 33-35, 37, 42, 43, 47, 48, 55, 58, 59, 62, 65, 70, 74-77, 87, 88, 91, 97, 104, 111-114, 137
   biological functions of 34
   expression 34, 34t
   inhibitors 1, 3, 26, 28f, 29, 29t, 31, 32, 36, 36t, 37t, 38, 38f, 41, 41t, 42-44, 46-49, 49fc, 52, 55, 61, 62t, 63, 64, 65fc, 65t, 68-70, 73, 76t, 82, 86, 87t, 88, 88t, 90, 92, 99, 100, 102, 112, 114f, 115, 123, 125, 126, 130f, 133
   adverse effects of 111
   development of 31
   effect of 91
   efficacy of 49, 60, 75
   first-generation 36, 38
   future of 78

nonselective 36
off-label uses of 96
oral 60, 76, 78, 122
rationale of 31, 90
role of 57
second-generation 36
selective 37
systemic 84
  side effects of 116
topical 42, 60, 76, 77t, 84, 122
use 126
work 75, 83
pathway, role of 25f, 106
receptor 21f, 113t
  types of 112f
signal transducer and activator of transcription
  pathway 6, 18, 19, 21, 24, 32, 35f, 47f, 48, 74, 82, 90, 111
  receptors 19, 96

K

Kaposi's varicella 115t
Keloid 98
Keratinocyte 75f, 82, 103
  apoptosis 83
Ketoconazole 62t
Kidney function test 122, 127
Klebsiella pneumoniae 13

L

Langerhans cells 82
Latent tuberculosis infection 127
Leptin 20
Leukemia 118
  inhibitory factor 112, 114
Leukocytoclastic angiitis, cutaneous 107
Leukocytoclastic vasculitis 98
  cutaneous 108
Lichen
  planopilaris 135, 139
  planus 19, 43, 90, 92, 98, 100, 135, 139
    hypertrophicus 100, 101
    immunopathogenesis 100
  sclerous et atrophicus 99
Lichenoid disorders 135
Lipid 121
  profile 127, 129

Lipoprotein
  high-density 115, 118, 121, 140
  low-density 115, 121, 140
Livedoid vasculopathy 139
Liver
  dysfunction 131
  enzyme elevations 139, 140
  function 115
    test 122, 127, 129, 140
Low blood cell count 115
Lower respiratory tract 119
  infections 139
Lung infections 119
Lupus
  erythematosus 98, 135, 139
  miliaris disseminatus faciei 99
Lymph node 4f
Lymphocyte 2f, 3, 10
Lymphoid tissue 14, 34
Lymphomas 118
Lymphopenia 61, 115, 139, 140

M

Macrophage 1, 19, 101
  activated disorders 12, 101
  inflammatory 34
Major adverse cardiovascular events 61, 66, 117, 126, 139
Major histocompatibility complex 3, 8, 47
Malignancy 78, 114, 115, 117, 118, 139
Mantoux test 127
Mast cells 103
Mediterranean fever 19
Membrane immunoglobulins 2
Mepolizumab 108
Methotrexate 38, 49, 50, 51f, 62, 101f
Microscopic polyangiitis 108
Migration inhibition factor 16
Minipulse, oral 46, 101, 108
Mitogen-activated protein kinase 21, 32
  pathways 32
Momelotinib 36
Monoclonal antibodies 26
Monocytes 34
Morbihan disease 98t
Morphea 98t, 135b
Multisystem autoimmune disease 106
Mycobacterium tuberculosis 7
Mycosis fungoides 112t

Myelofibrosis 26, 29, 41, 42
  high-risk
    primary 42
    secondary 42
  primary 38
Myeloproliferative disease 29t, 38
Myocardial infarction 117, 118

N

Naive T cells 3
Narrow-band ultraviolet B 76, 79
Nasopharyngitis 40, 66, 77, 115
Natural killer 2, 22, 134
  cell 1, 14, 34
    maturation 114
Nausea 40, 66, 115, 139
Necrobiosis lipoidica 42, 43, 99, 101, 135
Nemolizumab 104
Netherton syndrome 98
Neutropenia 61, 113, 115, 139, 140
Neutrophil 1, 19, 34
  extracellular traps 106
Neutrophilic disorders 139
Nonimmune cells 34
Nonmelanoma skin cancer 114, 115, 136, 139
Nonreceptor protein tyrosine kinases 137
Nonsegmental vitiligo 41
  treatment of 38
Non-ST elevation myocardial infarction 117
Nonsteroidal anti-inflammatory drugs 120, 125
Nuclear factor kappa B 20, 32, 34
Numerical rating scale score 91

O

Oclacitinib 37
Oncostatin M 24, 37, 102, 104, 112
Organic acid transporter 62
Osteomyelitis 119

P

Pacritinib 29, 37, 42
Pain, abdominal 139
Palmoplantar pustulosis 135*b*
Panniculitis 119
Papules 77*t*
Parthenium dermatitis 135*b*

Pathogen-associated molecular pattern receptors 2
Peficitinib 29, 36, 37, 42
Pemphigoid disorders 139
Pemphigus 135
Peritonitis 121
Pharmacokinetics 61, 134
Phosphodiesterase 57, 102
Phosphoinositide 21
Phosphorylation 23*f*
Placebo 122
Plantar keratoderma 99
Plaque psoriasis 29
  moderate-to-severe 29, 42
Platelet-rich plasma 99
Pneumocystis infections 119
Pneumonia 117
Polyangiitis 108
Polyarteritis nodosa 107
  cutaneous 135
Polycythemia
  primary 38
  vera 38, 41, 112
Polymorphic light eruption 99
Polymorphonuclear neutrophil 69
Povorcitinib 104
Progressive nodular histiocytosis 139
Progressive systemic sclerosis 99, 105
Prolactin 20, 24, 35
Protease-activated receptors 91
Protein
  acute phase 1
  inhibitors 23
Prurigo 139
  lesions 103
  nodularis 86, 87*t*, 92, 93, 103, 104, 105*f*, 135
  pathogenesis of 103*f*
Pruritic disorders 90
Pruritus 77, 90, 91
  chronic 92, 93
Psoriasis 30, 32, 36, 43, 68, 69*f*, 70, 92, 98, 117, 120, 126, 135, 139
  area and severity index 69, 135
  arthritis 31
  cutaneous 72*f*
  pathogenesis of 68
  treatment of 70*b*
  vulgaris 71*f*, 135
Psoriatic arthritis 29, 32, 41, 42, 70, 71*f*, 108, 111, 112, 135

Pulmonary embolism 118, 129, 130, 139
Pyelonephritis 117
Pyoderma gangrenosum 98*t*, 139

R

Randomized controlled trial 117, 128
Rash 139
Refractory acute graft-versus-host disease 41*t*
Refractory eczemas 135*b*
Renal disease, severe 126
Renal dysfunction, severe 125
Renal function tests 140
Resident memory T cells 74
Rheumatoid arthritis 26, 29, 32, 41, 42, 61, 111, 112, 126, 133
   moderate to severe 41, 42
Rheumatology 31, 141
Rifampicin 62*t*, 127
Risankizumab 70*b*
Ritlecitinib 30, 37, 40, 51, 76
   oral 78
Rituximab 108
Rodnan skin score, modified 106
Ropsacitinib 37, 76
Rosacea 99
   steroid-induced 99, 107
Ruxolitinib 29, 36, 38, 41, 43, 52, 60, 62, 65, 76-78, 82, 85, 92, 99, 102, 111, 112, 115, 119, 122

S

Salt scoring system 49
Sarcoidosis 99*t*, 101, 102, 135
Scabies 92*b*, 99*t*
Sclerosing disorders 139
Sclerosis, systemic 105, 135, 139
Secukinumab 70, 71*f*
Serlopitant 104
Shock, septic 119
Signal transducer and activator of transcription 20, 22, 24*f*, 25, 27, 33-35, 37, 58, 74, 75, 97, 102, 103, 112
   inhibitors 26, 28
Skin
   diseases 43*t*
   disorders, inflammatory 55
   neoplasms malignant 118
Small vessel vasculitis 108
Soft tissue neoplasms 118
Solcitinib 37

Spleen tyrosine kinase 99, 113
Staphylococcus aureus 56*f*
Stem cell factor 4
Stroke 115, 117
Sweet's syndrome 139
Systemic lupus erythematosus 26, 39, 106

T

T cell 3, 6, 16, 34
   autoreactive 106
   lymphoma, cutaneous 92
   receptor 2, 8
   regulatory 7, 16, 17, 177
   sensors of 2
T helper
   cells 7, 10, 12, 14, 60
   disorder 68
T lymphocyte 19, 105
   cytotoxic 3, 9
Tacrolimus 122
   topical 122
Takayasu arteritis 107, 108
Therapeutic paradigm 141
Thrombocythemia 140
   essential 38
   primary 38
Thrombocytopenia 113
Thromboembolic episodes 113
Thromboembolic events 115, 117, 118
Thromboembolism 39, 115, 126
Thrombopoietin 4, 20, 24, 35, 112-114
Thrombosis 139
Thymic stromal lymphopoietin 4, 14, 14*f*, 28, 48, 56, 82, 83, 91, 112, 138
Tildrakizumab 70
Tofacitinib 29, 30, 36-39, 41-43, 49, 50, 50*f*, 52, 58, 60, 62, 63*f*, 64-66, 72*f*, 76-78, 78*f*, 79, 84-88, 92, 93, 98*t*, 99, 100, 101*f*, 102, 104, 105*f*, 106, 112, 115, 119, 122, 126, 128, 133-136, 138*f*
   high dose of 118
   off-label uses of 135*b*
   oral 49, 76, 79*t*, 92, 102
   topical 85, 136
Toll-like receptor 6, 25, 33, 105
Tralokinumab 63, 64
Transaminitis 66
Transforming growth factor beta 5, 8, 11, 13, 17, 25, 27, 56, 69, 74
Transient receptor potential channels 92
Triamcinolone, topical 122

Trypanophobia 64
Tuberculosis 39, 52, 61, 66, 115, 119
  history of 125
Tumor necrosis factor 5, 6, 11, 32, 56, 69, 70, 74, 115, 135
  alpha 8, 13-15, 17, 32, 74, 87, 99, 100
  inhibitors 31, 102, 129
Tyrosine kinase 48, 58, 59, 70, 76, 83, 92, 96, 97, 99, 100, 112, 113

U

Ulcerative colitis 29, 32, 41, 42, 111, 112, 134
Ultraviolet 87
Upadacitinib 29, 30, 37, 40, 42, 52, 58, 61, 62, 64, 66, 82, 84, 86, 87, 99, 100, 104, 112, 115, 121, 133
Upper respiratory tract infection 40, 66, 115, 116, 139
Urinary tract infections 119, 139t
Urticaria 99t, 139t
Ustekinumab 70
Uveitis 31, 71f

V

Vaccines 128
Vascular endothelial growth factor 27
Vasculitides 108
Vasculitis 99, 107, 108
  cell-mediated 107
Vasculopathy 99, 107
Venous thromboembolism 114, 115, 129
VEXAS syndromes 139
Vitiligo 19, 29, 42, 43, 73, 76, 76t, 77t, 78, 99, 111, 112, 117, 135, 139
  etiopathogenesis of 73
  pathogenesis of 73, 74t, 75f
  repigmentation of 135
Vixarelimab 104t
Vomiting 115

W

Wegener granulomatosis 108
Weight gain 139
Wells criteria 130t

EU GSPR Authorised Reprsentative
Logos Europe, 9 rue Nicolas Poussin
1700, La Rochelle, France
Phone: +33 (0) 6 67 93 73 78
E-mail: contact@logoseurope.eu

www.ingramcontent.com/pod-product-compliance
Ingram Content Group UK Ltd.
Pitfield, Milton Keynes, MK11 3LW, UK
UKHW050428150426
5217IPUK00019B/1293